# WOMEN WHO WIN OVER DEPRESSION

We are all **WOW** women.

Luna Suhlyn Park

ISBN: 978-1-83556-101-0 PAPERBACK

ISBN: 978-1-83556-102-7 HARDBACK

ISBN: 978-1-83556-103-4 EBOOK

Book Design by HMDPUBLISHING

# DEDICATION

"I dedicate this book to my dearest family members and to all the cherished friends and colleagues I have met throughout my life.

Furthermore, I am grateful for being taught to always treat people with precious kindness and for the ability to share the love I have received."

John, Jun, Claire, Dounia, Yanni, Nacho, 洪哲彥, 李慧瑜, 洪詩蕙, 洪詩嘉, 陳彥伶, 譚皓瑋, Reina, Maho, Masayuki, Yuki, Kanda, Mamun, Isahq, Jung Min, Hak Su, Ah Hyun, Yun sung, Soon Jo, Soo Jeong, Eun Suk, An Jung, Hyun Jung, Sae Rom, Tintin.

# ABOUT THE AUTHOR

*Will this feeling ever go away? The pain in my stomach, the endless stream of anxious thoughts about tomorrow and the day after, perceptions of, "Will I be okay? Will I be alone and lonely forever? I've lost everything and everyone I love. What's the point of waking up tomorrow morning and the next day, and the next? I have no meaning, no purpose, no function in this world."*

*These haunting thoughts begin to seem even more real to me as the days pass. The days only go on getting darker and the sleepless nights longer and more draining. Sometimes a week feels like it passes slowly while other times, the days seem to pass so quickly. Either way, I feel like I'm just going through the motions...existing...but not living.*

*Will I be this way forever? Will this never go away?*

I don't recognise the person who wrote these words and conveyed these sentiments. Sometimes, I don't even know who that person is anymore, but not so long ago, this was *me*; these were my thoughts and feelings, and this was what my depression looked and felt like. It was a lifeless, dark place of despair, worthlessness, and doubt.

The person I was had disappeared or somehow morphed into an unrecognisable woman overcome with depression and anxiety, although I didn't realise at the time that it was indeed a severe case of these disorders. Depression was definitely the most prevalent, but the anxiety inevitably followed as I slowly watched my ability to function and my desire to live dwindle as the weeks and months passed me by. The world around me carried on, the people in it all going about their own daily business as normal. Their happy families and fantastic careers filled with promise carried on shining brightly. It seemed as if everywhere I looked, I saw these people—but I had absolutely no idea how to become one. I was lost. The world was leaving me behind.

Although I was at my lowest during this time, my inspiration for writing *Women Who Won Over Depression* was conceived. Everything I felt at the time seemed like the end, but the only semblance of some new beginning was my idea to somehow write a book.

I realized one day that if I were to survive this deep depression, I would need to share my story with others, specifically other women. I had to derive some type of meaning from this nightmare, and I also felt this intense desire to do what I could so others did not have to feel this way and live out their days wishing to be put out of their misery the same way I had. I thought, at the time, that the only source of meaning for my depression would be the creation of this book.

Little did I know that there would be so much more learning and growth for me. My profound fall was a precursor to the most significant years of my life. At the time, of course, I was unable to connect these crucial dots that I can now appreciate and look upon in gratitude and awe.

My story was similar to that of so many women, but hardships don't feel that way when you're alone and depressed. I thought I Was Only One who had to cope with the end of a relationship along with the death of my father during a tragic car accident. So, I thought my life was surely destined to be forever cursed when I lost three of my best friends to a dreadful natural disaster.

When I was in dire need of support, I was losing those closest to me, leaving me more alone and lonelier than I thought any human being could possibly endure. The life journey I'd imagined for myself completely vanished and I was left with a giant, blank void when I attempted to think of what kind of future I would have and what was to become of me. I lost count of the number of nights I spent crying to the point of exhaustion, but I do recall—despite the confusion I felt—that it lasted, rather severely, for a total of two years. *Two years*.

When I decided to write this book, I was still severely depressed, but I suppose there was a small dose of hope developing, like a tiny spring flower slowly blossoming, making its way over the tall, sharp blades of grass surrounding it. Other things were also flourishing, as I became much more compassionate toward the struggles of others, I judged less, and I listened more. My curiosity to study psychology and meditation grew intensely and, to my surprise, my compassion towards animals and the environment also developed. I looked into veganism not only for ethical reasons, but also for better physical and emotional health.

I began volunteering and attending workshops, courses, and seminars. I don't know if these activities helped my depression or if, after two years, my mind and body had simply opted out, deciding I had had enough—and the depression began to subside. And so, it did subside and left me much knowledge, renewed compassion, and empathy for others and for important causes, and with a strong desire to *never* keep this story to myself.

These few paragraphs are my story, but I decided that rather than go into chapter after chapter of my own experiences, I would tell the stories of some of the amazing women I had met, spoken to, and befriended. I would change all identifying information, but maintain the lesson behind their journeys, challenges, and triumphs. I would share the stories of these women through the new perspective and respect gained from falling into the depths of depression myself and managing to not only survive from what felt like a two-year coma, but awakening to a new life and a new *me*.

My depression provided me with a new start in life, allowed me to write a new story, and begin a new journey; it was a sort of rebirth within my same lifetime. The women I have had the honour to meet described a strikingly similar evolution of the self. The same sequence of events ensued. A seemingly predictable life, sudden tragedy, loss, a period of depression and confusion and finally, finding greater awareness and a new and more promising life journey.

I do always try to help as many women as possible whom I meet along my road to recovery. I always make time for them, whether I know them or whether I just happen to encounter them in my daily life.

It is with this open heart and spirit that I write this book and extend it to you. If it helps you, please pass your knowledge and sharing to another woman who needs help.

I hope my story and those of the women featured in this book can inspire you as you experience your own journey.

Luna Suhlyn Park.

11$^{th}$ March 2024.

# CONTENTS

# INTRODUCTION

I have not yet met a woman wholly untouched by depression. Is it even possible for a woman to go through life, to survive challenges, trying experiences and struggles, to reach success and achievement, without going through the hurdles and challenges that accompany depression?

It's my firm belief that depression is a condition that occurs during one or more periods in a woman's lifespan; an experience that women must fully embody to evolve, grow, and develop. It's as if you must survive depression before you can move on to achieve a higher, more centred, wiser version of yourself—a female self that is aware, present, and genuinely able to value yourself and your abilities.

Depression shows you, even in the hardest times, that change is part of life; that moments of hopelessness and despair eventually pass; and that the hardest times often come before new opportunities that will amaze you. You will look back at your most difficult moments in awe and even gratitude.

As women, we struggle with depression in a unique way, but we have so much in common in our experiences with depression. Just as we have so many feelings, emotions, and experiences in common, our ability to survive is also, in my view, similar and amazing. As a woman, you have a natural resilience within you. Difficult times often allow you to discover this resilience. Once you find it, you can become unstoppable in your journey towards discovering your inner strength.

Although depression can cause you to believe that you are completely alone in this situation, that the rest of the world is happy and satisfied and you are the only one suffering, the reality is that many women struggle and have struggled just like you.

I envision a united network where women who have overcome depression, along with those in recovery or in need of healing, can support each other in their shared journeys. *All* women experience this together. We realize this as we learn more about how depression is a part of a greater and more positive journey; a journey where we will find hope and the motivation to continue moving forward, no matter how difficult it can be at times. This same process can be true for you, too. You'll grow in respect, value, compassion, and love for yourself.

This book represents my thoughts about the struggles and successes of women, my observations and perceptions of women overcoming depression, and my beliefs about the key factors in coping with depression. I will share the stories of many women from different backgrounds, but with very similar journeys and stories of healing in common.

I want to encourage you, the reader, to find the courage to share your story.

Join me in this collective network of women that I imagine.

Will you?

Tell your story of current or past struggles, whether it be to one woman or many. Share the purpose that motivated you in continuing your journey so that you can instil hope in other women lacking the strength to continue. Sharing what you have learned makes your struggles more meaningful. Just imagine how great that will feel when you can take your wisdom—and how you made it through depression—to help another woman in her struggle! Challenges in life exist so you can grow and improve and so you can lend a hand to others along the way. I hope that you will receive this book as my way of reaching out to you in support, and my message to you is that you are not alone.

Believe me when I say you are stronger than you think; you can handle these emotions and conquer them; and you will emerge from depression with greater strength, courage, and resilience.

I encourage you to read this book with the belief that you will get through your current struggles. Once you do overcome these tough times, you can reach out to another woman in need.

# Chapter ONE

# WHAT IS DEPRESSION?

Can you remember the last time you saw a sad movie or news story that you considered "depressing"? In this case, the moment made you feel sad, discouraged, hopeless, or anxious. These thoughts and feelings of something being "depressing" are different from the experiences that occur in clinical depression—a very different state of depression.

Clinical depression, sometimes called Major Depressive Disorder or unipolar depression, is a severe mental health disorder that happens, at some point in life, to 20% of women and 12% of men. Depression is one of the most common reasons people seek mental health services. It is extremely common and a lot of times, these statistics and percentages are *under*estimated.

Just because depression affects so many people doesn't mean it can be treated easily like the common cold. Clinical depression is very serious; to the point that it can affect your ability to to everyday activities and live your life. Things like working, studying, eating, and sleeping can be affected and many people get this overall feeling that nothing in life is fun or enjoyable. Depression often prevents you from feeling any pleasure, even in all the things you used to enjoy and look forward to.

So what causes someone to feel this way? Believe it or not, scientific research hasn't discovered the answer to this question yet. Depression has existed for ages, but the exact cause remains a mystery. The fact that depression is felt very differently from person to person adds to the confusion. Research has concluded that depression occurs due to a combination of genetics, such as family history; a person's biology or biological factors; different things that a person can be exposed to in their environment, like different stressors; and psychological factors, such as the way a person thinks. Sometimes it just takes one of these factors to cause depression while other times depression can happen for a variety of reasons. Do you see why this disorder is such a mystery? Although it's important to know where depression comes from, it's even more important to understand different ways to treat it. Part of treatment is figuring out what's causing the depression so you can reduce or eliminate whatever is causing it. At the same time, it's important to avoid focusing too much on cause and instead, dedicate yourself to learning and developing ways to cope and practice those coping methods regularly.

## DIAGNOSING DEPRESSION

To diagnose clinical depression, you must meet a specific criteria that is found in the Diagnostic and Statistical Manual of Mental Disorder-5th edition (DSM 5; American Psychiatric Association, 2013). The DSM 5 is like the main reference for mental health disorders used by healthcare professionals to diagnose various mental health disorders. There is a specific list of nine symptoms and you must be affected by at least five of them most of the day, nearly every day for at least 2 weeks. The symptoms include:

- Depressed mood
- Diminished interest or pleasure in activities
- Significant weight loss or gain
- Inability to sleep or over-sleeping
- Psychomotor agitation (like pacing, nervous excitement, or wringing one's hands)
- Low energy or fatigue
- Feelings of worthlessness or guilt
- Decreased ability to think or concentrate
- Recurrent thoughts of death or suicidality, including suicidal thoughts with or without a specific plan, or suicide attempts.

In order for a person to be diagnosed with depression, these symptoms must cause significant distress in everyday life and the symptoms can't be due to anything else, like the effects of a medication or drug, a medical problem, or a different mental health problem that could be causing these symptoms. It's a bit complex, which is why it's important to be formally evaluated and diagnosed by a healthcare professional who is knowledgeable about depression.

# Chapter TWO

# WHEN DEPRESSION HITS UNEXPECTEDLY

*Susan is a 45-year-old mother of two children. For the past couple of weeks, she has noticed she's been more tired and less motivated than she has ever felt before. She feels like everything she does takes so much more effort and energy, even simple things like getting up in the mornings, taking a shower, making dinner, or cleaning up after the kids. Susan has also noticed her thinking is more negative than usual and sometimes, if she thinks of something sad, she starts crying suddenly.*

*Susan doesn't recall ever going through something like this. Her sleep has been irregular lately, and she's so much more irritable with others, almost like any little thing seems to bother her. Susan wonders if it could be stress that has her feeling this way or the fact that she doesn't take time to relax.*

*At the same time, she's not interested in reading or gardening like she used to and typically just watches TV when she has a few minutes to herself.*

Although women can experience depression anytime during their lives, Susan's story is a common example of the kind of depression you might experience in middle age. Many women describe it as happening suddenly. While Susan's story is an example of a mild form of depression, it can also occur severely and affect your ability to function or do even the simplest everyday tasks. If left untreated, depression can advance and lead you to believe that there must be something wrong with *you*.

It's important to view your depression as something that is separate from you; an issue outside of you. You are not your depression, and your depression isn't you. It's just a temporary state. By repeating to yourself that 'I suffer from depression,' you might be making the depression a part of who you are when it really is not. Instead, it's often more helpful to see depression as something that, yes, has changed how you feel, but is a temporary state. Just like any illness, with time, and with applying effective methods that help, the depression will soon pass. You might also consider telling yourself that you're suffering from depression *at the moment*.

See the difference?

The first way of thinking about it labels you as a victim of depression. You might then start to believe depression is permanently apart of you.

The second way of thinking about focus *the moment*—the current experience you are going through. You acknowledge your depression, but you understand that although it is difficult and painful in so many ways, it *is* temporary.

If you see your depression as a consequence of factors like stress, a major change in your life, disappointments, grief and loss, or financial difficulties, you will then be able to see it as something temporary and something that has happened *to* you—not something that *is* you.

Yes, even something depression has some sort of purpose. It is not a flaw you have or something abnormal about you. Many women describe it as an experience that made them slow down their lives and take a closer look at themselves. For many women, depression taught them many important life lessons. In many ways, it is a normal, human experience that can even turn out to be useful! But of course, they did not realise any of this until after the worst had passed. Life difficulties often help with seeing things more clearly.

## DEPRESSION IN MIDDLE AGE & BEYOND

Many women have similar symptoms, like the example of Susan, who had a more "classic case" of depression. However, your experience could be different since depression symptoms can vary from woman to woman. Below are some other examples of depression symptoms, particularly depression that occurs in the middle to late adulthood:

- Difficulty concentrating
- Difficulty in waking or getting up in the mornings
- Constant tiredness (and sleeping a lot)
- Memory problems, especially short-term memory
- Low self-esteem or feeling worthless
- Criticising yourself or putting yourself down
- Not wanting to answer the phone or feeling annoyed when the phone rings
- Preferring to stay home (if you typically enjoy going out)
- Loss of interest in socialising or being with loved ones or friends
- Feeling like you can't understand others or others can't understand you
- Loneliness (even if you have supportive people around you)
- Thinking of your future as hopeless (or believing nothing good awaits you in your future)
- Guilt feelings
- Thoughts of death, wanting to "disappear," or wishing to not awaken in the morning
- Decreasing personal hygiene (bathing, putting makeup on, dressing).

As you see, these symptoms are quite varied and can appear like you're just going through stress. This is why many women experience depression, but don't even know it until it gets worse. Depression can sometimes begin with mild symptoms until it suddenly gets so bad that you can no longer ignore it and you need to seek treatment.

You may find yourself wondering—why now? Why is this suddenly happening to you at this point of your life?

Well, there are so many reasons for depression to happen later on in life, even if you didn't experience it in your early adulthood years. Maybe you've experienced a major life change such as taking early retirement. Perhaps you have just begun menopause and your hormones have been thrown off balance, or you have another health issue. Maybe your grown-up children are enjoying their own lives more and more, and you are seeing them less. Or, maybe there's been *no* change, but you feel bored or dissatisfied with your life. Maybe you feel you have failed to achieve your goals. Sometimes, depression at this stage of your life could be related to a recent loss.

The reasons for depression occurring right now vary from person to person, but one thing is certain, and that's the fact that usually, depression is directing you to look at something important in your life that you need to pay attention to. Maybe it's something you've left unaddressed or neglected.

Depression is your mind and body telling you to look a little more closely because something within you needs healing. And when you think about it this way, doesn't it make sense that your depression is causing you to slow down and do less?

Your mind is telling you to take time out to heal.

## IS IT STRESS OR DEPRESSION?

If you've never struggled with depression before, you might think that it's just stress that's making you feel *different*. You might have no family history of depression and no reason that could explain the sudden symptoms you're feeling.

For these reasons, many women dismiss depression and believe it's *nothing*—just stress or *just a phase.*

So, how do you know if it is something more serious? How do you know that it's depression?

You can tell by how significantly the symptoms affect your life and your ability to function. A person going through extreme stress can appear a lot like a person with depression. When you're stressed, you're irritable and overwhelmed; you have difficulty concentrating and managing your everyday activities; and you may feel overwhelmed by everything or like you just want to give up.

People under a lot of stress physically *feel* very tired. Energy levels are almost always low. There may be stomach upsets, headaches, and muscular aches and pains. Your immunity may be lower, causing you to get coughs, colds, and other viruses more easily or more frequently than ever before. Stress can prevent you from falling or staying asleep at night and affect your appetite where you either eat too much or don't feel like eating at all.

These are symptoms typical of someone going through stress *or* someone with depression, but a primary factor differentiating the two is the quality of your *everyday functioning*. People who are stressed can typically still go about their lives, get things done, interact with family, friends, and loved ones, and even look forward to some time off or an activity they enjoy. They are stressed, sure, but they can *de-stress* after a long day, and eventually when the stressor is resolved, the person can get back to feeling like their normal self.

Depression is very different from the above; people with depression have difficulty going back to normal the way someone who is stressed can recover.

With depression, people still experience some or all of the symptoms above, but the symptoms are severe enough to affect their ability to live life. They can't just take a hot bath or go for a walk to "feel better."

This depth of despair and hopelessness can mean everyday activities like working, going to school, taking care of kids, cooking and cleaning, and interacting with family and friends become difficult or sometimes impossible. Many people with depression describe it as being under a dark cloud all the time. Even when you're smiling, you feel hopeless; you feel like crying; and you just want to stay away from everything and everyone. Perhaps you're missing work or school and even thinking of reasons to stay away. Maybe you suddenly need help around the house or with taking care of the kids. Perhaps your partner or a parent says you're 'letting yourself go,' not taking care of your appearance or hygiene, which might be unlike you. Or maybe you are under-performing at work, even if you love your job. Depression symptoms also tend to last long, sometimes a few weeks or more.

If you find any of these sounding familiar, you should know these are all signs of true depression rather than just stressors that will pass. Recognising this fact and these differences is very important because it can indicate that you may need some outside help. This is perfectly normal and to be expected.

So, depression can be triggered by stress, but it can also happen when there is no trigger. And, triggers *may* have caused the depression, but stress is not always going to be a trigger for you. Everyone's different. This can all be very confusing and frustrating when you're struggling with depression because it's hard to make sense of it and there is sometimes no way to predict it.

## SO, I HAVE DEPRESSION. NOW WHAT?

As with any life issue, it's important to become aware of it and admit to having a problem. When it comes to depression, you have to accept that you have it and understand that you need help. It is extremely important to avoid denying the existence of the problem.

It's natural to worry—as most people do—about acknowledging you have a mental health issue. This can bring on feelings of shame, especially in middle or late adulthood, after being emotionally healthy for the majority of your life! It seems easier to admit to physical illness than a mental health concern. Depression isn't something you can see or measure with blood tests or other physical exams. Therefore, you may fear you'll be considered 'crazy,' incompetent, or weak. You may feel there is shame in admitting to having depression and this may cause you to hide it and refuse help.

Well, here's the news! Depression is not something to be ashamed or embarrassed about, especially not nowadays. In fact, as many as one in three people will experience depression in their lifetime. Talk to people about depression openly, and you are likely to find many people say that they have it too, or they recovered from it, or they know someone suffering from it. So, don't be afraid to say how you feel. You'll be surprised just how many people feel the same way. This will immediately start to alleviate those feelings of shame that you might have.

You may feel that taking a positive approach and refusing to accept you have depression will be helpful. Although it is good to remain brave and fight against symptoms, doing this can become very stressful and can even worsen the depression. If you try to pretend it's not there, it could become a struggle for you as you try to act normal when you don't feel normal.

So, the first thing is to recognise the symptoms in yourself and acknowledge them.

From there, everything gets easier. Once you've taken the courageous step to admit you're struggling with depression, you can seek help. The most effective treatments are therapy and medication. When depression is mild, therapy alone can help, but if you're struggling with moderate to severe depression, sometimes therapy plus medication may be needed to get your symptoms under control. Again, try not to automatically dismiss the idea of taking medication, becoming one of those people who routinely say, 'I don't take tablets!' or believing that telling a therapist about your "problems" won't help. While taking any of these approaches may seem 'healthy' and brave, you might be rejecting what you actually need to get better. This could merely prolong your symptoms and your suffering.

Sometimes, depression may be caused by a chemical imbalance affecting the brain, so only medications will help, but it does not mean you will be stuck taking antidepressants forever. Think of depression as being like a physical injury. You would not treat a broken leg by saying, 'I won't bother with a plaster cast or surgery; I'll just wait for it to get better,' would you? Some forms of depression also won't just get better on their own. Let professionals help you to decide what to do; there are many treatments, and you can work with your doctor to find the best path to getting better—the route that's best for you.

# *Chapter* THREE

# ROMANCE, LOVE, & DEPRESSION

Love can make you feel more alive than you ever thought possible. However, when love goes wrong, it can bring about some of the most depressing times, leaving you feeling lonely, hopeless, and sad.

There eventually comes a time for most women when you realize that you have experienced enough heartbreak, hardship, and disappointment because of love. It is in this moment that you realize you need to evaluate your love relationships and let go of people who may be harmful to you and your life. It can be hard to make this kind of decision, but this is essential for your emotional health and wellbeing. The unfortunate truth is that some people are just not ready for a healthy relationship and may not have your best intentions in mind. Or, maybe they do but for whatever reason, you always seem to be at conflict with them.

Accepting that your partner is contributing to your depression is hard to face, especially if you desperately want the relationship to work. Here are some signs to watch out for to help you decide if the relationship can be saved or if your partner might be at least partly responsible for your inability to fully recover from depression.

## YOUR PARTNER DOESN'T SUPPORT YOUR GOALS

There's nothing worse than a partner who doesn't support your life goals. If someone is holding you back from reaching what you want in life, it won't be long before you start feeling depressed.

You and your partner may be interested in different things, but can still be working towards your own individual goals, like one of you getting promoted at work, running your first art show, or conquering the next wall at your climbing at the gym. If your partner is not goal-oriented like you are, it might feel like your partner is forcing you to choose between the relationship and what you want in life.

Even worse, in some cases, a non-goal-oriented person may become envious or jealous of the goal-oriented one and try to sabotage them. Some people might purposely try to stop you from achieving what you want most in life. If you see this happening, you probably need to get out of that relationship. Not only will it make you depressed, but it can also bring with it many other forms of controlling behaviours and abuse as the relationship progresses.

## YOU CAN'T CONNECT EMOTIONALLY

One of the best parts of being in a relationship is feeling like you can be vulnerable and honest with your feelings. The most reliable partners understand each other on a deep emotional level. So, when that emotional connection is not strong, or is missing entirely, it leaves both partners feeling confused and lost.

If you find you're much more willing to talk about your feelings than your partner, it may cause you to feel dissatisfied and misunderstood.

## YOUR PARTNER'S DEPRESSION MIGHT BE CONTAGIOUS

Is depression contagious? Researchers have tried to answer this question, and they've come up with extremely interesting results. One study looked at college roommates and found that students started experiencing depressive symptoms when a new depressed roommate moved in!

Even animal studies have shown that depression can be passed on to another person. Depression was induced in a group of rats, and when new happy rats were introduced to the cage, they quickly developed the same depressive symptoms as the group.

Of course, the more time you spend with someone who is depressed, the greater the chances are that you'll adopt a lot of their behaviours and even their feelings. This doesn't mean that you should leave your partner if they are depressed, but you have to be careful and ensure that you have good coping methods, supportive people in your life, and healthy activities that you can do to help alleviate the stress that comes from having a partner that is depressed. If you already struggle with depression, you must apply these strategies to make sure that your partner's depression does not worsen yours.

## YOUR PARTNER IS ABUSIVE

According to the research, it is likely for a partner to become depressed when the relationship is starting to become abusive. In fact, it's one of the main causes of depression in relationships.

Depression that results from partner abuse is also much more common than people realise, especially among women. Many cases of abuse experienced by women go unreported, and it's estimated that between 18% and 36% of all women have experienced some form of relationship abuse in their lifetimes. This abuse can be physical, verbal, or emotional.

Regardless of what form the abuse takes, you should look to loved ones for support and to experts outside of your relationship for advice and guidance on what to do to make sure that you are safe from harm.

## POOR COMMUNICATION

Poor (or lack of)_communication is one of the most common reasons for failed relationships. If you can't communicate with your partner, you might start to experience depression as a result. Whether one or both partners lacks communication skills, the relationship will likely suffer, contributing to depression.

## YOUR NEEDS HAVE CHANGED

Relationships are filled with many positive moments, particularly during the beginning stages. This period of time is also known as the 'honeymoon phase'. We often wish these moments could last forever, but people change and partners can become comfortable with each other as the years pass. This comfort can be positive, but it can negatively affect the relationship, too. Sometimes, one or both partners may eventually want to move on from the relationship and find another relationship with a different person.

Your partner may now have needs, priorities, and expectations different from those at the beginning of the relationship. Problems can happen when one or both partners can't meet the changing expectations of the other.

We can always compromise, can't we? An important question that both partners should ask themselves individually should be: "Can I change something so that I can compromise with my partner?" In a healthy relationship, partners must be willing to take turns *giving and taking*.

If both say yes, job done! If one says yes and one says no, then it's unfair to expect one person to do all the changing and compromising. You would need to look at couples counselling or some other form of working through things. And if both of you say no to making a compromise—then regrettably, it's all over unless you wish to live your life in a state of conflict, which is likely to make your depression much worse.

If you begin to grow apart from your partner, that's okay. Just because they seem like a great match in the past doesn't mean that you should hold onto someone who no longer meets your needs or has values different from your own.

## YOU FEEL 'STUCK' IN A FAILING RELATIONSHIP

Okay, so your relationship is making you depressed (or contributing to your depression). So why don't you leave?

Over the years, researchers have tried to figure out why people stay in unsatisfying relationships and they've come up with some interesting theories. Early studies claimed that couples stayed together because they thought they couldn't find anyone better, or that they were afraid of the uncertainty of separation. But modern researchers believe it's much more personal.

One new study suggested that people might stay together because their partner is exceptionally devoted or out of concern for each other's welfare. If your partner is saying things such as, "I can't live without you," or "You're the only good thing in my life," it can put a lot of pressure on you to keep them happy. You shouldn't feel like you have to accept certain behaviours or mistreatment if your relationship gets to a point where you are no longer happy.

You might also stay because you have a certain level of 'connection' and deep love for a person even though the relationship is filled with conflict. Maybe you just never found anyone you like being with as much as you do your partner, even if they are also the most difficult person to get along with! They probably think the same about you—and you both keep rebounding to each other following a separation. Each time is 'the very last time'—until you do it all again. Does that sound familiar?

Any of these reasons for staying with a partner when the relationship is dysfunctional—which simply means, it doesn't work—will likely contribute to one or both people developing depression. It's almost inevitable.

One reason why relationships do often end up in discord is if one partner is already depressed—i.e., when depression starts before relationship problems. If your partner is clinically depressed, there is nothing you can do to change that. Yes, you can provide comfort and support, but you cannot eliminate the depression. Your partner will re-experience depression unless he or she takes action and gets help. If your partner refuses, then it is possible that they see life very differently from you. They may believe that there is no point in trying and nothing to look forward to in life.

This type of negative thinking can lead to a very 'dysfunctional' relationship. There is help for this type of situation, such as couples therapy and your partner getting the appropriate help.

## INFIDELITY

One of the most difficult things to do when it comes to guiding others in self-development is helping a person who has gone through or has recently experienced being cheated on by a partner. There really are no words to console the feelings of anger, sadness, frustration, and fear felt by a woman who has found out her partner has been unfaithful.

In regards to depression, infidelity is by far a major contributor to the onset of depressive symptoms and in some cases, to a depressive episode. Even if you are one of the fortunate ones who has never really experienced depression before, being cheated on can certainly take you there, fast.

Another very difficult thing about giving 'advice' or feedback related to coping with infidelity is that fact that the best (and most commonly known) advice is that *time heals*. The problems with this advice is that it's pretty useless; useless because in the moments of pain and despair, a woman is usually not able to imagine any type of healing from the betrayal she has gone through. The idea that 'time heals' feels so distant that it almost seems unreal and completely unrealistic.

An interesting thing about infidelity is that women get better with practice. This fact is both depressing and also somewhat uplifting. What I mean is that once a woman has been betrayed once, she is able to understand that time really does heal. The pain of betrayal hurts just as much as the first time, maybe even more, but when you have experience, you know you will survive it and one day soon, you will be able to move on and smile again.

Could depression related to infidelity be prevented? Well, yes.... and no. We cannot see into the future and we cannot control other people, as much as we might try to in moments of desperation.

However, we can look out for warning signs of infidelity. This is a topic for another chapter...maybe even another book, but try to get to the point in your life where you don't see the warning signs looking backwards. Warning signs are meant to warn you, so if you see the signs, make sure you talk to your partner and if that's not possible, get help from a friend, a counsellor, a support group, or a religious leader in your community. Talk to someone so that you don't confirm that your partner is being unfaithful and then find yourself with no support available to you. Just having support and taking action to stand up for yourself can help prevent the depression that can come from infidelity.

# Chapter FOUR

# TRAUMATIC EXPERIENCES & DEPRESSION

When you understand how your brain reacts to trauma, you will be able to see how trauma impacts your physical body. So, the first thing we need to do is define trauma. What is trauma?

The real definition may surprise you.

Getting into a car accident or breaking an arm or a leg are considered traumatic experiences, but this is only a part of what it means to go through trauma. Your reaction to the event is another key part. Then there is your instinct for survival. Certain parts of the brain react to traumatic life events and this determines how a trauma can develop.

Here's one example.

Let's imagine Anna was abused when she was a child. But she has gone through counselling and she feels perfectly fine; in fact, she always felt 'perfectly fine.' Anna feels that she came through her trauma with no leftover damage, unlike her sister who was also abused and tends to cry at the slightest thing, has an anger problem, and a fear of men. Anna just went for counselling because her sister went along and wanted moral support.

Because Anna has no 'feeling' of being traumatised, she must be okay, right?

Well, no.

Anna doesn't even realise that she may well be carrying trauma with her, and that it resurfaces even when she is not realising it. She does not realise she is displaying signs of trauma in small ways and that these signs affect many things she does, and certainly her interactions with other people and in her relationships.

When the brain processes trauma, or any adverse event where the person feels helpless, the  instinct to protect yourself from harm emerges. It turns out that the key to understanding trauma is finding out how the brain responds to that feeling of helplessness. So, in Anna's case, she perhaps feels fine until something triggers her feelings of helplessness. She may go on feeling 'fine' until this very thing happens. Anna will then find she is unable to be in control, suddenly bringing out her vulnerability.

When your brain experiences any event that has a negative consequence and causes you to feel helpless, your survival strategies of 'fight or flight' are activated. The 'fight or flight' response is a stress response that happens automatically without you having to do anything. Signals are sent from your brain to your body (and vice versa) alerting you to either 'fight' off the threat you are facing or escape (i.e., 'flee') the threat.

These reactions exist to protect you from harm and help you survive the event, which your brain perceives as potentially life-threatening.

It is beneficial to have this 'fight or flight' response that allows us to take action to protect ourselves from harm. But the trouble with trauma is that the human brain has a way of learning to associate many things—even events much later on in life—with the actual trauma that happened to you long ago, and then re-start the process of 'fight or flight' over and over and over, often years after the real threat has passed.

It's important to understand that this happens to all of us, all the time. The brain and the body have an excellent way of remembering past trauma. Your brain/body remembers in order to protect you from similar threats happening to you again.

So, it seems like the next question must be, what can you do to break the cycle of trauma? The answer is complex, or actually, applying strategies and solutions to heal from trauma is complex.

A good place to start and a strategy that has helped numerous women is to begin by observing your thoughts when you experience feelings like anxiety, worry, sadness, and anger, among numerous other emotions. The emotions will be different for anyone, but these are just a few examples of the common ones related to past trauma experiences.

When you place yourself in the role of the observer, you are creating a separation between you and your anxious, fearful, and/or sad thoughts. This separation is how you slowly begin to realize that your trauma-related thoughts are a production of your brain and body meant to keep you safe from future harm. However, your brain/body sometimes perceives non-threatening things as threatening. This is where the separation of you and your thoughts is effective because you will begin to notice that your mind is constantly reacting to non-threatening things. And, the best part about this strategy is that once you realize you can observe your own thoughts, you will also see that if you can think and observe at the same time, this means that you, the observer, are not the same being or the same entity as the "person" creating the thoughts. It might take some time to understand this concept if you haven't read or heard about mindfulness, but consider this concept for a moment: If you can observe something, anything, then it must mean that you are not the same as the "thing" you are observing. You are something else, outside of that observation—that thought. With time, you will learn more and discover who You are; that being that is so much more than the being that is producing the anxious or depressing thoughts.

So, practice this observing exercise. Observe your thoughts when you are stressed, anxious, sad, lonely, fearful, worried, or angry. Imagine yourself stepping outside of your own mind and watching those thoughts, like a movie playing on a big screen. Try to avoid getting upset with yourself over having negative or dysfunctional thoughts. Be gentle with yourself as you engage in this process. You've been through a lot and that's why those thoughts are there. Plus, you are a survivor and those thoughts are there because you have survived. Watch the thoughts, watch the content of the thoughts, and then watch the thoughts as they pass.

# Chapter FIVE

# DEPRESSION AND SENSITIVITY

There is a distinct relationship between depression and being 'highly sensitive.' A highly sensitive person (also known as HSP) is someone who feels physical, emotional, or mental reactions to certain life situations much more strongly than the "average" person. These individuals are also known as empaths, which is a term that comes from having a high degree of empathy.

High sensitivity comes from a person's way of thinking and interpreting events in their environment, so this can be a complicated and often lonely way of living when you're 'over-sensitive.' Being a HSP is also frequently misunderstood by other people who are less sensitive.

Sensitive behaviour comes from many direct and indirect factors, like people around you, the environments you spend time in, and your thoughts and emotions.

Anyone can become sensitive at one time or another, but everyone handles this feeling in different ways. People who are highly sensitive experience deeper emotions in response to particular situations. These situations can be overwhelming and cause a sensitive person to feel isolated from others.

Many HSPs prefer to be alone due to a fear of being exposed to more situations where their sensitivity can be triggered. Isolation can become an excellent solution because it gives the person time to get over any emotions they feel. HSPs have a deeper understanding and thought process of situations others might overlook. Being highly sensitive is something that may be evident since childhood, but tends to develop further with age.

Even though HSPs are "different," they often find ways to deal with it. A key factor in coping is being aware that you have this quality because this will help you evaluate situations where you find that you feel hurt, offended, or misunderstood so you can re-think these situations a bit and better cope with your feelings.

## ABOUT HIGHLY SENSITIVE PEOPLE

Here are three certainties everybody should know about highly sensitive, empathic individuals:

1. Being highly sensitive is a fairly common thing. About fifteen to twenty percent of people in the world have the quality.
2. Being highly sensitive is also called Sensory Preparing Sensitivity (SPS), which is a quality that can be seen in brain images. These individuals have other "abilities" too, aside from just being highly sensitive. Being highly sensitive also means that you are able to perceive or sense the feelings and intentions of others better than the average person.
3. High sensitivity is associated with introversion. Many introverts are also highly sensitive. It's also no coincidence that depression is believed to occur more commonly among introverted people (and HSPs, too). This is believed to occur because extroverted people cope with feelings that could potentially lead to depression by expressing their feelings outward, towards other people and/or situations. Extroverts will tend to talk to people about themselves and their feelings or in some cases, even lash out in anger on someone else in order to "feel better" and release these emotions. Introverts, on the other hand, are more likely to keep feelings to themselves and spend time alone if something is bothering them. This isolation can lead to the onset or worsening of depression.

Being highly sensitive can bring on both strengths and weaknesses. For instance, very sensitive individuals will, in general, be compassionate, intuitive, and very mindful of the needs of others, to such an extent that many do well in professions as advisors, guides, specialists, artists, and journalists. However, HSPs can also become overwhelmed and suffer frequent burnouts, particularly from absorbing the emotions of the people around them. Noisy, crowded, or fast-paced environments can be much too overstimulating for an HSP.

HSPs can sometimes be mistaken as being too self-absorbed or anti-social. This, of course, is not the case. The reality is quite the opposite.

## QUALITIES OF SENSITIVE INDIVIDUALS

If you are wondering whether you're considered highly sensitive, consider these signs.

If people close to you often say you feel things "too" deeply, you're "too" easily offended, or that you're "overly dramatic," you're likely an HSP. In reality, you aren't "too" much of anything. You simply have a unique quality.

Empathy is another quality of many HSPs. These individuals tend to be very good at sensing the feelings of others. They are careful with their words and actions because they do not wish to hurt anyone or cause harm. The downside to this is that sometimes, HSPs can be too careful to the point that they may be too self-conscious due to their concern about what others will think of them. They are highly aware of the needs of others and they are very helpful to other people.

For an HSP, empathy isn't just understanding somebody else's feelings. These individuals can often feel the emotions of others even when other people don't communicate what they feel. This is one of the reasons these individuals are known as empaths; because they take on the emotions of others as their own.

HSPs are very good at perceiving social signs or signals the average person may overlook because they are highly sensitive to everything that is going on in their environment, and this includes other people's thoughts, feelings, and needs. HSPs will often sense sounds, discrete changes, scents, or tastes that others don't pick up. This is what often causes these individuals to become overly stimulated.

If you are an HSP, remember just one thing above all: You are a normal person who just happens to have these unique qualities and characteristics. Other people who are not highly sensitive have other personal strengths, as well as flaws and weaknesses of their own.

## THE WORLD NEEDS MORE COMPASSIONATE INDIVIDUALS

HSPs can succeed in the world; there is no doubt about that. If you're a compassionate individual, this means that you're very familiar with the feelings of being overpowered, stressed, and over-burdened. For numerous HSPs, these overwhelming feelings can become a huge burden to carry. Some may stress that something is "broken" inside them, while others feel excluded by the many non-sensitive people around them. However, remember that your sensitivity is much more of a positive quality than it is a negative one.

Being very sensitive is quite extraordinary, so if you are exceptionally sensitive, the world needs more individuals just like you. Being caring and attentive to the feelings and needs of others will ultimately bring greater joy in life. Many HSPs who have embraced their highly sensitive nature will often report that there are far more benefits that disadvantages to having these traits. So long as you are aware of your highly sensitive nature, you can act to ensure that being an HSP benefits you, helping you learn more about yourself and your abilities.

# Chapter SIX

# HOW TO THRIVE AS A RECOVERING DEPRESSIVE

People who have depression often see themselves as weak. To appear this way to others or for the depressed person to feel this way isn't a personal defect; it is just a normal reaction of a truly depressed person. It isn't the individual who is broken; it is society's understanding of depression that is the problem.

There is nothing wrong with communicating your real emotions, even if you are going through severe depression. People who are passionate are those who contribute to a caring and thoughtful world. Never be embarrassed to show your emotions and shed tears.

With that said, being a depressive person can become confusing at times. You might ask yourself:

Why do I get overpowered by emotions that other people seem to deal with easily?

Why do I get so hurt by negative comments from others and take these comments so personally?

Why do I overthink things that other people seem to dismiss easily?

Oftentimes, people with depression are missing certain defenses that others appear to have.

You might attempt to hide this about yourself, but it still hurts and you struggle to let go of things that hurt you. Maybe you tend to think about these things over and over again.

"You're overthinking things. You're too sensitive. You should be stronger than this!" You have probably heard these times of comments from others many times. This leaves you pondering what might be the matter with you. You wonder if there are other people who think and feel the same way you do. Wouldn't it be wonderful to hear the words, "You feel that? So, do I!"

Many people with depression feel disconnected from others. They feel misunderstood and abnormal and don't know why. They don't understand that there is an explanation for why they are different.

There are many famous figures that struggled with depression or were highly emotional. Albert Einstein, Martin Luther King, and Steve Jobs all became depressed at some point in their lives. This means that suffering from depression will not stop you from succeeding in your life and living a life of meaning, like these influential people did.

However, when you don't understand how to deal with your depression, you end putting too much pressure on yourself your focus is on trying to be "normal" like other people. You feel like your goal must be to function the way "normal" people do, or even function better than them. The problem with this is that it could make your depression worse.

If you identify with any of this, here are ten ways you, as a recovering depressive, can quit fighting against depression and instead, begin to flourish.

## STOP HUNTING FOR SOMEONE OR SOMETHING TO FIX YOU

For many women, when depression strikes, we immediately try to problem-solving so we can find an explanation, and a solution for the sadness, lack of energy, the crying, and all the other symptoms that stop you from living and enjoying life.

Sometimes, you might find that depression causes you to become impatient, especially if you're not able to do all the daily tasks you're used to doing. Your family, friends, or loved ones might keeping asking you what's wrong, why you don't smile anymore, or why you seem so unhappy with yourself.

Some women explore solutions like dietary changes, hormone therapy, vitamins, supplements, and herbs while others use methods like life coaching, reading self-development books, meditation, or even psychotherapy. These activities are all excellent options to explore, but it is important to understand that there is no single solution that will fix or eliminate your depression. There isn't even two or more solutions that will get rid of depression for you. Even antidepressants, which often take up to six weeks to work, won't get rid of depression entirely.

The reason that there is nothing out there that will fix you is because recovering from depression is a process. Depression cannot be fixed by treating the wound, putting a bandage on it, and then waiting for it to heal. The process of healing is a little more complex and takes time. Many people believe that time itself will heal depression.

It takes self-reflection, it takes caring for yourself, and it takes mental and physical rest. Sure, it's important to be proactive and search for treatments, but always remember that there comes a point where you must do what you can, and then let go of control. Let go of trying to control your depression and heal it as quickly as possible.

Many women want their depression to get "fixed" so they can go back to their old life, their habits, their relationships, and their routine. The problem with this is that oftentimes, it is one or more areas of your life that may have brought about your depression in the first place. Now, you want to get better quickly so you can go back to your old life. Do you see the problem with this? Do you see how going back to the same routine might cause you to experience depression again and again?

Stop hunting for someone or something to fix you and most importantly, avoid rushing the process. True healing is achieved with time.

## LET YOURSELF KNOW YOU'RE NOT FAKE

Many highly-accomplished individuals experience a lot of distress and anxiety thinking that other people may discover their depression—that their 'weakness' will me made known to others. People often prefer to admit to having a physical illness before revealing that they have depression. Although women tend to be more open about talking about depression compared to men, we still struggle; we try to remain brave and strong and avoid admitting to any emotional weakness.

Regardless of how you view depression, it's likely that you're aware of the social stigma related to it. Stigma is what causes many people to hide how they feel. This does not mean you are being fake or dishonest. It simply means that you are trying to survive in your environment. Sadly, when we admit to a weakness, we risk being judged by other people.

If you are struggling to hide your depression, or if you're frustrated by trying to feel "normal," it helps to focus on your strengths, accomplishments, and positive qualities. This enables you to be your genuine self. When you focus on your positive traits, you are also building your self-esteem, which not only helps you be your genuine self, but it also helps in alleviating depression.

## SEEK OUT LIKE-MINDED PEOPLE

Positive social support is critical if you struggle with depression. It helps to spend time with people who are open and accepting of themselves and others. These genuine people comprehend what it means when you feel isolated, and they can offer first-hand experiences and advice. Simply being around such people and the emotional support you derive from this will help you to better cope with your depression. Seeking out like-minded people helps you to feel less alone in a world where you may often feel like you have to hide your emotions and be brave. You can *let go* around like-minded people

People recovering from depression often acknowledge they have depression and know that other people see it. In case you're feeling unsupported or misunderstood, seek out a sensitive and friendly mentor, a tutor, a group, or peers who understand you and will support you in it.

## RELISH THE CONCEALED ENERGY IN CIRCUMSTANCES

As a depressive person, you need to learn to recognise the negative (but not over-examine it), and then release it.

Immerse yourself in positive activities and circumstances that make you feel better, or possibly give you a liberating feeling. This is especially important if you have to spend time in situations where you cannot be your true self, like at work, in social settings, and even around family and friends. These could be circumstances where you may feel you must hide aspects of yourself and conceal your depression. For these reasons, you should make sure to also surround yourself among things you enjoy and are passionate about and in surroundings where you can speak your mind and show 'weaknesses' freely without fear of judgment. For many people, one of the primary reasons depression can get much worse is if they must constantly pretend that it's not there.

## TREAT YOURSELF WITH SYMPATHY

As a person coping with depression, you're most likely your own greatest critic. You push yourself hard, and after that, you criticise yourself if you don't succeed. You treat yourself in ways you would never treat others.

Being aware of negative thoughts and feelings is the foundation to developing self-empathy. You shouldn't disregard your negative or depressive feelings. Thinking, and sometimes thinking too much, is one of your gifts, so why not make use of it? Take control by observing your own thoughts, but without judgment, and afterwards moving onto feelings that trigger kinder and more nurturing feelings. From that "feel better" place, you're ready to live positively.

People recovering from depression must show themselves the same kindness and empathy as they give to others. It might feel childish or vain at first; however, it's most certainly not. If your basic internal voice is making you feel worse, answer back with self-generosity as this is the "antivenom."

## CREATE BOUNDARIES THAT AREN'T RIDDLED WITH EMOTION

We live in a culture that advocates "take a painkiller and push on." This philosophy is often more emphasized than sensitivity and self-care. We grow up hearing that pain is what leads to the results we want; that survival is for the strong and that life isn't fair and we must get used to it.

We appreciate individuals who show toughness to overcome difficulties.

As a depressive individual, you might automatically think that you have to persist through challenges, or if you can't, you must show courage against them. You protect yourself from emotional pain through avoidance and other strategies like creating drama in your life to distract you, working all the time, using liquor or medications, or becoming involved in toxic relationships.

You commit to avoiding emotions by overthinking everything, always trying to control everything around you. Then, you get upset with yourself about how you should avoid overthinking every little thing. This becomes an endless cycle.

Recovering depressive individuals show delicate yet firm boundaries. If you struggle to put your own needs first, something that is often challenging for a depressed individual, practice saying "no," or cutting out alone time to re-energise.

## LISTEN TO WHAT YOUR BODY SAYS

Many depressed individuals figure out how to disregard the messages their bodies are sending them. They ignore them to avoid feeling overwhelmed, or they worry more out others' needs than their own. Oftentimes, women with depression ignore important emotional and physical signals because they have gotten used to minimizing their own feelings for so long that it becomes normal and natural for them.

Doing this causes you to abandon yourself.

When you don't listen to your body and your emotions, you can either become over-animated and then exhausted. This is similar to starting a workout program and then exercising excessively to the point that you're so exhausted that you have to take a break for several days.

Recovering depressives are very aware of the physical sensations in their bodies; they acknowledge that it's not always positive news, yet they trust their bodies to direct them. If you tend to escape your emotions or deny them entirely, figure out how to perceive your body's obvious signs of overstimulation. Do you feel exhausted, overwhelmed, angry, frustrated, or irritable at times? These could be signals that you need to rest and recuperate, spend time alone, and reconnect with the places and/or things that bring you happiness and tranquillity. Practice listening to your body rather than putting off your self-care for 'later' or 'tomorrow.' This is especially important if you have a history of putting your needs aside on a constant basis. It's important for you to discover that there is likely a direct link between your tendency to not listen to your body and your depression. Once you see this, you can break this connection by doing the exact opposite and rather than ignoring your needs or putting your needs off for later, you will know to pause and tend to your self-care.

## MAKE USE OF HEALTHY HABITS

In the long run, failing to take care of yourself will affect you physically and emotionally. Overwhelming hours at work, followed by hard perspiration sessions at the gym and taking care of your home and family can leave you with little time for yourself.

If you go to excessive lengths and put too much strain on your body, not resting in between, you risk lots of ailments. However, if you overprotect yourself, your energies go unexpressed and unused; that, likewise, can prompt your wellbeing to be put into jeopardy.

Recovering depressives practice habits that support them. In the event that you're battling with health or money issues, organise activities that support these parts of your life, (for example, more rest and alone time), and stay home for a while if you're aware you've been overdoing it at the gym or otherwise pushing the boundaries too much.

## DON'T IGNORE IT; GET HELP

After a lifetime of being overloaded by stimuli, it becomes natural to you to dismiss how you feel and try to ignore your depression. You find you can block out certain feelings, for instance, so you can convince yourself you don't care at all. You minimize or try to ignore extreme emotions, both good or bad, so you can avoid any extremes. You smother feelings to get a break from everything and everyone around you.

This self-defence instrument may trick your consciousness, yet it doesn't trick your sensitive body. This will gradually affect your wellbeing, your connections, your focus, each part of your life—creating strain until your body cannot take it anymore.

Let go of the need for control.

When you release your hold on control, you free the gifts of sensitivity that have been lost to you: sympathy, imagination, and increased satisfaction, to name a few. What's more, you enable your actual potential to show itself.

Remember that the way to recover from depression, more than anything else, is to perceive that it's alright to be depressed—with all its difficulties and qualities.

Identify if you are, indeed, hiding or denying your depression and purposely refocus your energy and the realistic options available to you. Remain genuine and true to yourself.

# Chapter SEVEN

# PRENATAL & POSTPARTUM DEPRESSION AND THE POSTPARTUM BLUES

*Last night, I was watching a show on BBC Africa. It was emotional, as the story was about a county in Kenya where there has been a case of 73 young men committing suicide. Many of these suicides are linked to depression, which made me think of my struggle with depression and how things could have turned out differently for me, should I not have decided to make a positive change in my life.*

*As a mother of two boys, life can become tough at times. In 2015 when I was pregnant with my second child, I had a condition called hyperemesis, a condition where I couldn't eat, and I couldn't drink anything. Because of this, I became severely dehydrated and suffered from malnutrition.*

*When I finally went to see the doctor with my husband, I told the doctor what I was going through. The doctor's response was, "Oh, you know, a lot of women go through nausea and the motions of pregnancy. You have several options to help you get better. You can take acupuncture or ginger or wait it out. You'll see, it will soon be over."*

*I remember my husband telling the doctor that what I was feeling was different. It was not your normal morning sickness. He told the doctor that he felt I was severely depressed.*

*When I heard him say that, I was shocked and immediately denied the fact.*

*But as my husband insisted, I was referred to the main psychiatric hospital where my case would be evaluated. From there, both my physical and mental health began deteriorating, and I found myself having suicidal thoughts. I was aware that my thoughts and feelings were a combination of both situational, environmental, and hormonal, and to be honest, it was just crazy. I was in a very, very dark place.*

*As my evaluation was completed in the psychiatric hospital, I was taken to suicide watch. While there, I needed to do a nutritional evaluation where it was found that I needed nutritional therapy, which involved a natural gastric tube that went through my nose and into my stomach. Although it scared me to the core, if I think back to it, that intervention saved me and my baby's life.*

*But in the process of all that, I developed serious prenatal depression. And the prenatal depression slipped into postnatal depression when my son was born. I didn't know what I was going through, but I remember feeling suffocated. I remember being in a dark place, which is a common symptom of depression.*

*Another symptom that I experienced was severe anxiety in the form of self-consciousness. I would have extremely sweaty palms, and I was always fatigued. That led me to have a loss of appetite yet again. With the loss of appetite, I had difficulty sleeping. I would be lying in bed, and my heart would race. I just wanted to get out of my head because it felt like I was in too deep.*

*When you're depressed, you're trapped inside your head. You want to get out of your head. Thus, when you lie down to go to sleep, you find yourself running around in your head, trying to find a way to escape. It's like a machine that keeps churning out thoughts. And usually, those thoughts are very, negative self-deprecating thoughts that question your self-worth and your self-esteem. All this leads to insomnia. I had insomnia to the point that I needed to take sleeping aids.*

*Funny enough, before I became depressed, I was an extrovert and someone who thrived socially. Coming from Kenya, I've always been around people as we share a collectivist culture. But when I was depressed, I found myself becoming a recluse. I pulled out, and I felt like an introvert. I made all kinds of excuses not to socialise.*

*I remember my husband always trying to push me to go out, but my mind always told me that my friends were going to say that I was boring and not fun to be around.*

*And that's the thing; depression is deceiving. Depression creates doubt and tells you that you're not worthy, and you're boring. You have issues, and it messes with your perception of things. It messes with your reality.*

*And so, I found myself always trying to make an excuse to be alone; always making an excuse for why I did not need to socialise. I would feel guilty, yet I didn't do anything about it.*

*As time wore on, I realised that I had to find acceptance in the fact that I was going through something with which I needed help. If I had cancer, I wouldn't think twice about going for chemotherapy. If I were involved in an accident, I wouldn't think twice about having physical therapy. So why do I need to think twice about seeking help if I have depression, anxiety, or panic attacks?*

## PRENATAL DEPRESSION

We mostly hear about postpartum depression, the type of depression women can experience shortly after giving birth. However, prenatal depression is not discussed nearly as much. The hormonal shifts and changes that occur at the onset of pregnancy can be quite significant for many women. Changes in your energy level, taste and preferences, mood, sleeping habits, appetite, and physical appearance all occur due to the effects of hormones. Mental health can change significantly during pregnancy. Afterall, hormonal changes affect brain chemicals, which can contribute to depression, anxiety, and other emotional concerns among *all* people: Women, men; pregnant, or not pregnant.

Prenatal depression symptoms are very similar to those of traditional depression: sadness, loss of interest, feelings of emptiness, difficulty concentrating, irritability, crying spells, changes in sleep schedule and appetite, low energy, and guilt feelings. The tricky thing about prenatal depression is that many women attribute it simply to the *typical* symptoms of pregnancy. They believe they should feel this way because that's how pregnancy is *supposed* to feel. The truth is that although women should expect some pregnancy symptoms, depression is not considered a "typical" or "normal" part of the prenatal period.

Many women are skeptical to take antidepressant medication during pregnancy and this is understandable. But, this should not mean that you should keep these symptoms to yourself and avoid talking about it. A significant part of any type of depression treatment, whether during pregnancy or not, is talking to someone about it and sharing any fears or concerns you may have. Even if prenatal depression is not a "normal" part of the pregnancy process, it is still something that many women go through. Your doctor can suggest many different treatment strategies that can prepare you for, and allow you to enjoy, the remainder of your pregnancy.

## POSTPARTUM DEPRESSION

Postpartum depression is the most common form of depression associated with women after childbirth. It can range from mild cases, where the woman can recover after interventions and treatment, to more severe cases that can make it difficult for the mother to care for herself and her newborn child.

Just like prenatal depression, postpartum depression can occur due to the changes and shifts in hormones after childbirth. These hormonal changes affect brain chemicals and can cause symptoms of depression. Women who have postpartum depression can sometimes report anxiety symptoms and extreme exhaustion, too. Some women even experience psychotic symptoms during postpartum depressive episodes. What is likely the worst symptom of all is the feelings of guilt that mother's with postpartum depression experience, as they feel unable to properly care for their child. This guilt is, in itself, part of the depression, but is particularly difficult for mother's to cope with as they try to fulfill their new role.

As with all types of depression, it is critical for mother's to normalize what they are feeling. I am not saying that it is normal to have postpartum depression, but it is very common among mother's shortly after childbirth and it is something that women do not have control over. Normalizing the symptoms and feelings the woman is experiencing helps to eliminate some of the pressure she feels to "get better" quickly so she can care for her baby. Recovery from postpartum depression cannot be rushed in this way. The mother needs support from others, intensive treatment, and self-care in order to return to her regular level of functioning. Sometimes, with time, symptoms can decrease or disappear, once the woman's hormonal levels have returned to normal. However, women should never wait for the symptoms to resolve and should always speak to their doctor and seek treatment throughout the process.

Education on postpartum depression helps mother's to understand those guilt feelings and realize that the feelings are there because they want to be the best mother they can be for their child. This type of education is really a benefit to any mother as their child grows and parenting demands increase. Women often feel an immense pressure to do everything right and be the best parent, but it is important to keep in mind that perfection is not the goal. Caring for yourself and growing in your own self-love is one of the best gifts you can give to your child, as this will make you a more effective and loving parent.

It's important to keep in mind that although cases where a mother with postpartum depression has thoughts of harming her newborn child are very rare, they do occur in some cases. These symptoms are out of the mother's control and are due to problems with brain and body chemistry. There is no shame in reporting to your doctor or any emergency service that you feel this way or are having these thoughts. It is actually quite courageous to do so. There is treatment available for you and options to help you get through this tough time.

## POSTPARTUM BLUES

The postpartum blues, also known as the "baby blues," are a very common condition that occurs among women just after childbirth. This state of "blues" includes feelings of sadness, worry, and low energy or fatigue that often results from the constant care that a newborn needs, leaving the mother feeling exhausted and stressed.

The postpartum blues often resolve on its own and lasts anywhere between one to two weeks. Although women do not always need treatment for the postpartum blues, it is important to talk to your doctor, identify the condition, and take action to minimize stress and get help or support. Your baby will require all of your time and attention at first, so getting support is critical. If you don't have any type of childcare options available to you, there are groups that your doctor can tell you about where you can meet with and talk to other mother's going through similar stressors. This type of support group can help you connect with other women and share some of your own feelings and experiences. You can take your newborn with you, too. Getting together with a support group is often considered an effective way to alleviate depression.

# Chapter EIGHT

# MAINTAINING YOUR IDENTITY AS A WOMAN

You likely always knew that being a mother meant you had to fulfil many roles, but you probably never realised how much it could consume your whole identity, did you?

Your role as a mother isn't made up of simply *one* job or a single responsibility. Many titles are given to mothers to describe their roles and duties or the "*types*" of mums they are. Maybe you were/are known as a *working mum*, balancing a career, a home, and children. Or maybe you are a *stay-at-home mum*, putting your life on pause to take care of your home and children. Then there are *single mums*; *mums in blended families*; *mums who travel for work*; or even mums who have had life circumstances that separated them from their children.

All these titles still label you as a mum first and foremost. They are roles unique to women and assumed with pride and much gratitude.

And while there's nothing wrong in that, and while you have every reason to be proud of being a mum, you should also hold onto your individuality.

Remember, even before you became a mother, you might have been a wife and a partner first, so you've already been through several transitions.

Regardless of the *mum type* you belong to, once you started a family, your identity changed completely from being just you and the woman you are, to becoming a mum, a wife, and most likely, the primary caretaker of the household. Your role became that of *the one who does it all in the home* and like most mothers and wives, you likely fulfilled your role with commitment and enthusiasm even during the most difficult moments.

You may find that giving all your energy and dedication into this role, this new and permanent identity, the woman you were before children and family is put aside and, in many cases, it disappears.

You may even believe you must say goodbye to that woman forever because how can you keep that identity while also tending to your many duties as a mother? You might end up feeling guilty for taking time for yourself due to all the demands you have in your life. And when you find that identity returning, even if only briefly, you immediately feel you'll be judged for not being good enough or available enough for your children and family. Maybe you'll judge *yourself* a little bit, too.

The truth is, mothers have to put forth a lot of effort in order to maintain their identity as women. The loss of identity is at least partly caused by stereotypes and pressures from society, from family members, from other mothers, or it might also come from the pressure and demands mums place on themselves.

However, keeping the identity of *you*, the *woman*—not just you as a mother and wife—is so important for your health, your well-being, and for maintaining your quality of life. Keeping this identity alive will help you to enjoy your role as a mum more than ever and allow you to give the best of yourself to your family.

If your children are already grown and independent, rediscovering your identity apart from the identity of *Mum* will provide so much more meaning and purpose, allowing you to experience greater joy and gratitude.

Finding your identity is a big task because you might have to go back several years or maybe decades when you first became a wife and mother! So, let's go step-by-step, focusing instead on strategies you can implement to rediscover this important part of who you are.

The best way to create habits and new and healthy behaviours is to build upon the personal strengths you have and develop new skills that will take you closer to your goal. However, you must set the intention, the *goal*, to rediscover your identity and to commit to working towards this new journey in your life where greater growth and opportunities lie ahead for you.

## HOW LOSING YOUR IDENTITY IS ASSOCIATED WITH DEPRESSION

So, your identity as an individual, as a woman, has slipped through your fingers to the point that maybe you don't even refer to yourself as '*I*' anymore. It's only '*we*' now because you have selflessly devoted yourself, entirely and wholeheartedly, to your role as a wife and mother. A big part of you loves this role, but does the role love you back?

With every good intention, you've devoted yourself to your husband and family, leaving behind many—or all—of your interests and likes, the things that made you feel whole and alive. Now and then, amid your role as a wife and mum, you recall the old days when you used to devote time to your passions and interests, but you had to put those things aside to fulfil your new roles.

As is the law of life, change happens. Children grow older and increasingly independent. Your relationship with your husband may change, or, as is the case with more than half of marriages, the relationship may, sadly, dissolve. Too many women experience these very difficult, but also very common, scenarios in life where sometimes, all of a sudden, they realise they gave all of themselves and now are left with nothing. They expected their role as wife and mother to always stay the same and provide them with a sense of comfort and stability. We all know, however, that change is inevitable—so when things do change, and you have spent years, sometimes decades, building an identity, what happens to you when the inevitable occurs and things do change?

Depression kicks in for many because they have based their whole identity on the lives of others and not on their own needs. They realise they are left with no real meaning or purpose.

## STARTING WITH A SELF-EVALUATION

If you are reading this, you are probably already aware you've lost touch with your identity. In your journey towards rediscovering it, it is important to understand there will be challenges that prevent progress on this new path.

So, what sort of challenges?

Challenges often come in the form of excuses that take you back to engaging in old behaviours, for example, "I'm too busy," or "My kids need me." Guilt is also a barrier that can stop you along this journey and can lead to making excuses.

Many women wish to rediscover their identities, but get distracted by believing they do not have time for themselves; that self-care is a luxury they don't deserve; that their children need them; or that they are neglecting their duty as a mother by investing time in themselves. Remember that these challenges are just guilt—guilt that is maintained by unrealistic expectations placed on you by society. Everyone deserves an identity and a personal life.

Think about whether the pressures from society causes you to believe unrealistic ideals and stereotypes about mums. If you want to stick to your commitment to rediscovering your identity, you must evaluate your thoughts and beliefs and challenge the ones that make you feel guilty for nurturing your identity or make you feel you need to fit a 'mould' or expectation.

For instance, a common negative belief many mums have—and which can contribute to feelings of guilt—is the idea that spending time doing something they enjoy is selfish or self-serving and instead, they should be dedicating all that time to their kids. Many feel guilty for going to a workout class or sitting for an hour reading a good book. Catching a film without the kids or going out to a restaurant with friends is not what they are supposed to be doing—or is it?

If you have any of these negative beliefs stemming from guilt or stereotypes about being a mum, it's important to become aware of them, question their reality, and challenge them. Ask yourself why it's wrong for you to engage in self-care? Who said that being a mum means you must neglect time for yourself to do some of the activities you enjoy? And most importantly, consider whether you can give your all to your children and your family if you neglect taking care of yourself by doing so? How beneficial is that to your children?

Could losing your identity negatively affect your relationship with your family and interfere with your ability to fulfil all of your roles as a mum effectively? And, could being happier, and having more balance in your life, enhance your relationships with your kids and your ability to care for them?

It's important to be aware of your own negative beliefs that may interfere with your journey towards establishing your identity. Creating goals and developing specific reasons for staying on this journey will help you remain on track despite any challenges that may get in the way.

## GOAL SETTING

If you want to get your identity back and strengthen it more than ever before, goal setting is an important first step. Discovering your identity means different things for different women. For some women, getting their identity back means going back to school and continuing or completing a degree, while others may decide they want to go back to work or volunteer.

Many women have lost contact with social relationships and friendships, and they want to join a local club, committee, or some organisation to meet new people and develop new friendships. Maybe for you, getting your identity back means something as simple as taking on a new hobby or having your *me time* a couple of days weekly, where you set aside time to relax or do something you enjoy.

Whatever "getting your identity back" means for you, make sure to set specific goals to achieve that identity. Imagine what you will look like, feel like, and how you'll act when you've reconnected with your identity and when you begin to invest quality time in yourself.

Setting a specific schedule of the activities you'll start doing and *writing this schedule down* is best if you want this plan to be effective. Goal settings prevents those moments where you might procrastinate or when you try to convince yourself that you have other "more important" things to do. Plus, writing down goals symbolises a commitment you're making to yourself. Set a reminder on your smartphone or post a written reminder somewhere you're sure to see it. Tell your family and partner about your new goals and encourage them to ask you about them, which will ensure you also look forward to updating your loved ones on your progress.

Now, bear in mind that achieving the goals you set will take time, so avoid putting too much pressure on yourself or expect too much, especially right at the start.

It takes the average person approximately thirty days to develop a new habit, so set yourself these reminders for the next four weeks until it becomes a solid habit in your life to participate in these identity-discovering activities.

It is also helpful to identify any potential issues that may slow down your progress towards your goals. Imagine how your child falls ill just as you're about to embark on your first evening class, and you need to stay home with her. Don't feel defeated or say, "Well, I knew this could never work!" because you're just blighting your possibilities. Instead, accept the circumstance and then re-book your class or find a new commitment. Each challenge you have is only that: one challenge. That's life. Your time will come, so stay determined and avoid chastising yourself if you have to cancel new commitments to take care of your personal ones.

However, at the same time, try and put these commitments—to yourself—first. Will your daughter suffer if Daddy stays home with her when she's sick, instead of you? How about Granny? It's natural to leap into Wonder Woman role, motivated and spurred by guilt when really, the job can be taken on quite competently by someone else.

It's like that first day when your child starts school. You hate it, right? But it has to be done. Sometimes, the best and most unexpected things can happen when you challenge yourself and move forward towards something new. Being a great mum doesn't mean being there 100% of the time, and it also benefits children when they get to spend time with others; they gain self-esteem and a sense of achievement.

## IDENTIFYING YOUR STRENGTHS

When you spend many years identifying as a mum and a wife, your life duties revolve around caretaking. It's common to put your identity aside and to forget about your strengths, particularly those unrelated to your role as a wife and mother. Don't underestimate the importance of keeping these strengths at the forefront of your mind, especially on your journey of rediscovering your identity.

Your strengths are your skills and abilities, the things you enjoy doing, and the tasks and topics in life about which you are most passionate. It is important to have a clear picture of what your strengths are, from which you will derive much of your self-esteem and self-confidence. By nurturing your strengths and becoming involved in things you are passionate about, you can find true meaning and happiness.

Rediscovering your identity can seem like an overwhelming accomplishment. It's common to think, *where do I start*? Especially if it's been so long since you've connected with yourself and your innermost being and it's why identifying your strengths is such an important step on this journey. It breaks down this big task of self-discovery into something smaller and more manageable. Plus, when you start to let yourself remember those tasks and activities you're good at, and when you remember what you're most passionate about, you will find how you will immediately experience a positive and hopeful feeling, like your life can be fun and exciting again, you are not stagnated, and you have many amazing opportunities to look forward to in your future.

Make a list of all your strengths and abilities. Think of things you know you are good at or enjoy and avoid listing anything of which others have told you that you're good, as it's all about you—what you want, and what will fulfil you. Other people may see you from their perspective and biases. This activity, though, is about *how you see yourself* and the things you know, deep down, are what you love and connect with most. Forget everyone else and put yourself first for a change!

# Chapter NINE

# LETTING GO OF "BRAVERY"

Women are assigned many stereotypes, but a primary one is that we are emotional. We are also known to have the ability to communicate and express our thoughts and feelings more easily than men. Women are also given more "permission" to cry compared to men—because *that's what women do*. However, given all these stereotypes about women, do you really express and show your emotions when and how you should? Do you validate your thoughts, feelings, and emotions show yourself compassion?

Many women go through life keeping a façade in place. Emotions are often left unexpressed for a long time, sometimes for years or even a lifetime. As women, we often do this so we can put others first.

We believe we must be strong, patient, understanding, tolerant, and forgiving. Interestingly, women are called emotional, yet our ability to endure some of the most difficult emotions—with the utmost courage—is astonishing.

When you do, finally, express your emotions, it is often because you've held on so long that you can't contain your feelings any longer. Emotions then come pouring out.

You might hold back emotion quite often for this exact reason. You know that once you allow those feelings out, the emotions can be overwhelming and intense. So, you might feel you're protecting yourself by trying to avoid emotions—especially the most intense ones. You continue to cope with the many trials of life—love, loss, children, marriage, career, responsibilities, and your numerous other life demands.

Other reasons you may hold back emotion can be due to the fact that other people—those around you and even loved ones—may not validate your emotions. This can lead you to prefer tp keep your emotions to yourself. Society teaches us to be critical of ourselves if we show any type of emotional struggle, as this is considered a "weakness." Showing emotion is, unfortunately, sometimes considered weak.

When weakness is not tolerated, you may that fear others will be intolerant of your emotions too; that is if you dare expose even the slightest bit of feeling!

Have you ever confessed to someone at work or even to a close friend or family member that you're just not having a good day or that you feel sad, down, worried, anxious, and depressed? If you haven't done this recently, try it out, just as an experiment and observe their response.

If you're lucky enough to receive an empathic and compassionate response, where the person encourages you to express yourself and your feelings, then you are very fortunate, indeed, and that person is likely very special.

However, you might find that the person responds in in a way that minimises your emotion, with statements such as, "Stay positive!" or, "You'll be fine." In some cases, you might end up having to hear all about how that person feels, the horrible day they had, and how stressed out they are. Sometimes people may not know how to respond when you share your problems, so they "respond" by telling you about their own troubles!

Here you are, trying to share with another person that you're feeling down or are having a personal problem and the response is far from supportive or motivating! The result could often be you fulfilling the role of a therapist for that person.

Although this does not occur in every case, as a general rule, people fear displays of emotion. Many people who have considered committing the tragic act of suicide, had previously made attempts to talk to someone about it.

Imagine, in such a severe state, being told to keep a stiff upper lip or to try to *make the best* of the situation. In such a moment of despair, it is critical to show the person in distress some compassion and empathy. We all need it at one point or another, and in cases where the person is experiencing severe depression or more serious concerns, showing compassion and empathy could save someone's life.

Expecting this level of compassion and empathy from others, however, might be mostly unrealistic. Sometimes, your own problems and emotions are too much for you to handle, so how can you deal with the tribulations of others? So, you ask yourself: *"How can I expect from others what I also struggle to deliver myself?"*

Some people may not be great listeners—an issue that can also be due to being overwhelmed with personal problems. However, one thing's for sure: You can always learn to listen to yourself.

It's important to show yourself this compassion when you are struggling emotionally. Rely on yourself to be honest, open, and genuine with your own feelings and give yourself the compassion and empathy you need. You can be your own source of validation and motivation. Learn to encourage and inspire yourself when you need it most. This is a skill that takes much practise because most people are not taught to treat themselves with compassion and care. We often live our lives believing also that when others approve of us, this means we are worthy. That isn't so. In fact, only your own opinion of yourself is what really matters in most cases.

In your journey towards overcoming depression and healing from emotional wounds you sustained along the way, allow yourself to express your emotions without fear or avoidance. When you hold back sadness, frustration, loneliness, despair, and anger, you will only internalise those feelings. An accumulation of emotion and tension develops from keeping those feelings within you rather than expressing them.

It might take some time to get used to openly expressing yourself because for many people, we get accustomed to holding back emotion since childhood when we are told not to cry or we are scolded for becoming upset or showing feelings. When you get rejected or criticised for showing emotion, you learn to avoid showing your feelings because no one wants to feel embarrassed, humiliated, or rejected, especially when it comes to something so personal.

Try practising expressing your emotions and being your own source of empathy, compassion, and support. Think about emotions you've been keeping stowed away for a long time. For some people, learning to express emotion means crying and allowing others to see you cry without shame or embarrassment—without concerning yourself with what others will think of you. For others, it's about showing their fears—whether its fear of abandonment or fear that they miss someone for whom they care. Some refuse to show weakness or any indication they need help from someone else. Discover your own hidden emotions and gradually make an effort to express them.

Identify those emotions and maybe write them down. Then, consider how you can begin to uncover them. Set your emotions free and you will see how this will help you heal from depression. You can gradually become more genuine with yourself and with others.

Most importantly, validate your emotions as true, real, and worthy. Tell yourself it's your right to feel those emotions, and you are strong for being able to acknowledge them. Depression, fear, and many other emotions can worsen from hiding or minimising your own emotions. You will become stronger from expressing emotion and learning to comfort and support yourself.

## THE HEALING POWERS OF CRYING

Crying is a very healthy expression of emotion. It lowers blood pressure and eliminates stress hormones and other chemicals from the body. If these bodily hormones and chemicals are not released, it can increase negative emotions. Aside from these physical benefits, crying provides a major relief from stress, and some people even say if they are worried or anxious, the act of crying decreases or even alleviates those feelings. That's another reason why expressing emotion is so critical.

You can probably now see why holding back emotion and not allowing yourself to *feel* and experience sorrow (without fear or avoidance) can have harmful effects on your body and emotions, especially in the long term.

The story of Gloria (see below) is a perfect example that comes to mind, illustrating the importance of being comfortable with the vulnerability that comes with showing your emotion.

To me, Gloria was an example of a strong woman. But Gloria wasn't born strong and resilient. She had gone through her fair share of defeat, failures, and even trauma and loss. Gloria learned to be resilient and strong because she once considered herself very weak and vulnerable. As a child she was teased by her peers and even her older siblings, often being called a "cry baby."

"Cry baby, cry baby." They teased her constantly until one day, Gloria was sent to the Principal's office for the first time in her life, at age 11, for pulling another girl's hair. She fought back after being teased by a classmate because she had been holding back her anger for so long.

This event was rather significant in Gloria's life because after this incident, she never let anyone see her cry again. Ever.

It was as if Gloria found some source of inner strength and although she was never physically aggressive with anyone after that incident in school with her classmate, she learned to defend herself verbally. However, she never cried. As Gloria grew into her adolescent years, she became a "tough girl." She was told other names unfortunately given to women who are strong and assertive. Gloria didn't care and even seemed to like it. She was a smart young woman and quickly learned to defend herself without showing any fear.

In adulthood, Gloria worked in sales and became very successful in her career. She worked in a setting where emotions and feelings were discouraged. In fact, being emotionally vulnerable was seen as a personal weakness in her industry. Gloria had no problem with this, and she fitted right in with the work culture.

She was able to be compassionate by being a bit gentler with close family and childhood friends, but with anyone else, she was always considered "serious, strong Gloria." Some would even say she had no heart.

Things changed for Gloria one day when she learned that an earthquake had struck in a vacation destination close to her hometown and killed her two best friends. Gloria was devastated, and at first, the shock left her feeling no emotion at all. She went about her daily life in this non emotional state for a long time. Gloria took a leave of absence from work because she found she couldn't focus, had difficulty sleeping, and was often feeling physically ill.

With time, Gloria developed much guilt; the truth was, she and her two best friends had planned to go to that vacation town together, but Gloria had cancelled at the last minute because she had to work. Then the earthquake struck, and suddenly, her friends were gone.

Gloria valued her friendships very much, as she was only able to be vulnerable with a select group of people and these two friends were among those she felt she could trust and with whom she could be herself. These were very cherished relationships to Gloria, and suddenly, they were taken from her.

Several months later, Gloria was unable to recover from her guilt, grief, and loss, and it was affecting her work more severely. Her sales performance declined, so before she found herself at risk of losing her job. This is when she decided to see a counsellor. After several weeks of therapy, she and the counsellor concluded Gloria was struggling with grieving the loss of her friends due to her inability to express emotion healthily.

Since Gloria was called a cry baby as a child, she developed a very strong defence against being vulnerable and emotional. As a younger child, Gloria was able to cry when something bothered her, but as she grew into adolescence and adulthood, she never cried. It took her six weeks of therapy to finally be able to cry about the death of her friends. She hadn't even been able to let out her grief during the memorial service after her friends had passed.

The years of holding back emotion and being unable to express emotion healthily finally affected Gloria when she had to grieve the death of people she loves. Gloria learned a very important lesson—that those who are truly strong can be vulnerable too.

When Gloria returned to work after nearly a year of emotional struggles and therapy, she hugged all of her co-workers and even cried at work, something she would have never done before. She finally healed from emotional wounds she carried since childhood and learned to express herself and her feelings openly and genuinely. After crying at work on her first day back, Gloria was able to continue with her day feeling relieved and with a sense of freedom, like a great weight had been lifted from her shoulders.

Now, she could be her genuine self. She remained a strong, intelligent woman always, but now the confidence and inner peace she had developed allowed her to experience life with greater joy.

# Chapter TEN

# MINDFULNESS FOR DEPRESSION

Some people hear the word *mindfulness* and immediately think meditation is not for them. If you feel this way, you're not alone. Many people find it difficult to meditate and often give up after the first few attempts.

Mindfulness, however, is not just about the traditional type of meditation where you have to sit still, breathe, and clear your mind. Meditation is just one of the many practices of mindfulness; certainly not the only one.

Mindfulness or *being mindful* involves being fully present in the here and now. As a wife and mother, with numerous responsibilities and stressors, you might find your thoughts are constantly on events that have happened in the past, or you are often worried about what may happen in the future. If you struggle with depression and/or anxiety, your thoughts will often tend to go in either of these two directions.

When your thoughts are past-focused, you may become saddened at things that may not have turned out how you wanted or guilty over things you can't control. Those things are in the past; what can you do about them now? Why waste time now, revisiting the past? We know the answers to these questions, but applying these principles is a different story.

When your thoughts are future-focused, you might worry a lot about outcomes or if decisions you make now could have negative consequences later on. While some degree of future planning is healthy and necessary, avoid the trap of over-planning and then feeling life's a failure when it takes a different curve! Over-planning can also cause you to avoid risk—and to miss out on many aspects of a fun and healthy life. Both of these scenarios can contribute to depression.

Mindfulness exercises help you practice keeping your mind and your thoughts, in the here and now. People able to maintain this presence in the moment tend to be happier and more satisfied in life. Why? Because you can enjoy life as it happens. *The only moment you have any control over is right now, this very moment.*

## ACTIVE MINDFULNESS

If you haven't been able to succeed at traditional meditation methods where you sit down with your legs crossed, and clear your mind as you take deep breaths, then *active mindfulness* might be a great way to get the benefits of mindfulness.

Active mindfulness is not only fun but also, you might find it will reveal so much about your everyday activities and *where* your mind is as you do daily tasks.

Think, for instance, about the last time you stood at your kitchen sink, washing dishes.

So, you are standing there, washing a huge pile of dishes after dinner. Think about where your mind goes during those twenty minutes or so.

What did you think about the last time you washed dishes?

Or, the last time you loaded your washing machine or brushed your teeth?

You might be thinking about how one of your kids has a school project due in two days and how they haven't even started on it, or what you will say to your boss when you have to ask for a day off next week to make it to your doctor's appointment.

Then you might worry about the results of the bloodwork you had done recently. And then there's that awful doctor's receptionist who's so rude; you hate going in the practice. Or, your mind might drift to an argument you had with your husband about finances, and that might lead you to think about the bills you haven't paid yet this month, and about all the terrible *what-ifs* that may come to pass if you can't improve your cash flow.

Before you know it, the whole time you spent washing dishes just went by as you imagined the many problems and stressors from days in the past and days ahead. But, the reality is that these events either already happened—so you can't do anything to change the outcomes—or, they may never occur at all.

Now think about another scenario, instead.

Imagine you are washing the dishes, and you place your attention on how the warm water feels on your hands and the sensation on your skin as the water streams down and touches your skin. Then you move your focus to the fresh scent of the dish soap and the sound the water makes as it hits the base of the sink. Watch as you soap each dish and swirl the sponge around in circles and then rinse the suds off with water. Notice all that's happening as you spend time doing this chore.

It may seem unusual to notice your actions while washing dishes because it's something you do automatically and doesn't require any real concentration. It may even seem like a waste of time thinking about the dish suds! Surely, you tell yourself, it's more productive to think through the problems of life?

Well, no—it really is not more productive. You see, the whole purpose of mindfulness is to focus on exactly what you are doing, *at the moment*, regardless of what you are doping. When you bring your thoughts to the here and now, you won't be thinking about your son's science project, your health, the argument you had with your husband, your boss, or the bills. You are fully focused on right now and giving yourself a break from stress, worry, and trying to problem-solve constantly. If we allow it, our minds will get stressed, worry, and problem-solve all the time.

And does it truly help you when you get stressed over things while you wash the dishes or load the laundry? No, it doesn't. So, give yourself a break and indulge in mindfulness.

You will enjoy improved mental health in many areas, such as your focus, attention, memory, improved sleep, less worry and sadness, and a more positive mood.

## MINDFULNESS AND BEING GENTLE WITH YOURSELF

In practising simple mindfulness exercises, working on *self-compassion* is extremely important.

Mindfulness involves not just quieting the mind from thoughts and images; it's also about practising *acceptance* and *patience* so that when those thoughts do arise as you are practising mindfulness, you learn to accept them, observe the thoughts, and *let them go*.

You probably tell yourself a lot of self-defeating and negative messages; maybe on a daily basis and several times daily. Mindfulness helps you become aware of your own negative thinking so you can then practice self-acceptance and self-compassion, pushing away negativity.

Often, you might not even be aware you're telling yourself these negative messages, but when you purposefully engage in mindfulness—where the goal is to focus on the here and now—you will realise the places your mind goes where you judge and criticise yourself, sometimes harshly.

Even in the act of mindfulness, some people find that if their mind drifts to thoughts about the past or the future, they begin to engage in criticising themselves for being unable to accomplish the task at hand. For example, they may believe they don't have enough self-control or are too anxious or stressed to meditate or practice mindfulness exercises.

If you find this happens to you, just know that thoughts will inevitably come to your mind during mindfulness exercises—it's normal, especially when you're first starting and aren't that experienced in practice yet.

In mindfulness, you must observe the thought, whatever it is, whether it's a negative thought about yourself, a worry, a fear of what's to come, or the replaying of events that happened yesterday or days, weeks, months, or years in the past. Accept the thoughts and then imagine them passing by you like the wind carrying a leaf in the air and blowing it away, or ocean waves washing up to the shore and then retreating into the vast ocean. Even if positive or neutral thoughts come to you as you are practicing mindfulness or even if you get distracted, do the same thing: Accept the thought and then let it pass.

With repetition, you will begin to engage in this process automatically and find yourself living in the present more and more. You will also find that you will be more forgiving and empathic towards yourself—and towards others, too. Mindfulness will teach you to accept yourself and events around you. By allowing negative thoughts to pass by, you'll begin to realise *you are not your thoughts*—a significant learning experience gained from mindfulness. Your thoughts are automatic, even reflexive creations of your mind. You are separate because you are the observer of your thoughts.

## WHY YOU SHOULD LEAVE THE PAST BEHIND FOR GOOD

I talk to so many women who have been through difficult times, disappointments, failures, profound losses, and betrayals of all sorts.

I very often hear how they blame themselves; I hear their anger, frustration, and how they lost hope in their ability to change their life course. They spend a lot of time thinking about how different their lives would have been if they would have made better life decisions.

These women are unable to let go of the past. As they talk about and replay past events, their emotional reaction is the same as if the event were still occurring. The fear, the depression, or the guilt all remain the same. Healing cannot occur in this state.

Why are we all so often afraid of letting go of the past and of releasing those memories that keep the past alive? I can't speak to the experiences of others because there are so many individual differences when it comes to difficulties with leaving negative experiences behind, but I feel a primary component could be the inability to forgive oneself for mistakes, errors, poor decisions, or any other supposed fault related to the past event.

Now, of course, I am not referring to people who are clinically traumatised and develop more serious symptoms. What I am referring to is when you feel guilt, self-blame, and persist in an inability to move on from a past you regret. You see, by forgiving yourself and understanding and accepting that you are not perfect—that no one succeeds all the time—you are more likely to be able to let go of the past. Letting go will free you and allow you to live in the moment.

Part of forgiving yourself is accepting you were a different person in your past. You had a different mindset; you had less life experience, you were younger, your feelings and emotions were different, and—probably what is most important—you cannot predict the future and see the possible outcomes of your actions and decisions. Learning from experiences—especially the negative ones—helps you to make better decisions and improve yourself,.

Let go of your need to achieve perfection, forgive yourself, and allow the mistakes of your past to remain part of your life *history*. Your past has no role in your journey forward.

Leave it behind you and only extract what you learned from this important part of your history.

When life is running smoothly and easily, we don't really learn that much. We get comfortable when there are no challenges.

When life gets difficult, and when things happen that you don't want, you gain knowledge, wisdom, and courage. You also discover the resilience you have. It may take time to recognise it, but you do grow from adversity and challenges.

You would never have the opportunity to see this side of yourself during the times your life is running smoothly.

Consider taking another look at your past and the emotional scars you've sustained from the experiences you've overcome. What do you see if you look at your past from a place of acceptance and forgiveness? What did you endure? What did you *survive*? Consider how you can be grateful for your past. This is how you know you have grown from adversity—when you can be glad that you went through difficult times because of how much you gained from them.

# Chapter ELEVEN
# ACCEPTANCE

Do you accept yourself fully, with all of your flaws and weaknesses? Do you feel you acknowledge and accept your strengths and positive traits? Do you accept events that happen to you in your life, even if you dislike them or didn't want them to happen? Acceptance was one of the most cherished journeys for Mary Anne, a woman I knew for many years.

I will tell Mary Anne's story of how acceptance changed everything for her and set her on a path of achieving greater courage, as well as amazing and new opportunities.

As an adolescent, Mary Anne appeared confident and outgoing. She was very sociable, charismatic, and friendly, but beneath these outward characteristics, another side of her was insecure, hyper-aware of what others would think of her—especially her peers—and very self-critical, particularly about her physical appearance.

As Mary Anne grew older, into her twenties, she noticed a change in her where she cared less about what others thought of her, and focused more on her future, her career, and her close relationships with her partner, family, and friends. The opinions of those who were not close to Mary Anne didn't seem to matter as much and, for the first time in her life, she felt greater confidence and acceptance of herself. Mary Anne even felt satisfied with her physical appearance, which was something she'd struggled with for so many years.

As she entered her thirties, Mary Anne experienced a new sort of transition and change. She still had that confidence she'd developed in her twenties, but as the years went by, she *lived* more and had more experiences. There were good and happy times, but also sad and dark moments of stress, challenges, and failures, both personally and professionally. Mary Anne felt these experiences with family, love, career, and life, in general, started to affect her emotionally, particularly her self-confidence. Then, Mary Anne experienced depression for the first time in her life.

It took Mary Anne several years to get through her depression, and there were moments when she felt completely hopeless and worthless, believing she would never feel better from the sadness, worries, and fears she had developed. She felt her life was over and often wished she could disappear. Mary Anne didn't see any hope for herself and felt she had no options. She only thought of her past mistakes and constantly worried about what would become of her future. She was obsessed with maintaining perfection in her life and when things were suddenly *not perfect* and when she experienced depression, she was unable to cope.

Mary Anne was trapped between these two realities, and it drove her crazy.

However, with time, she eventually grew tired of depression and sadness. It was exhausting to be so sad, afraid, and worried about the future all the time. She never got a break from these feelings and she became so physically and emotionally tired from the sadness and worrying.

This led to her sudden decision one day to live her life and not think or worry anymore—about the past or the future; about possible consequences or outcomes. She decided she was not going to try to "solve" anything. Mary Anne let go of trying to control her depression and how she felt.

She had quit her previous job where she was earning a very good income and had taken a less stressful and lower-paying job instead. Although she didn't make much money, she nonetheless decided she didn't care. She stopped becoming stressed about her income or her future; she stopped worrying about when her depression would "get better."

Mary Anne grew so tired of the constant pressure she was putting on herself—pressure that she realized was likely making her sick—that she decided to give up all effort, *live her life*, and accept her current circumstances, even if that meant accepting her depression. So, she did. She accepted her depression, her worries, her fears—everything. Mary Anne allowed herself to feel unwell. She gave herself space.

In taking this step, Mary Anne realised the obsession she had with planning and with maintaining perfection in her life—whether it was at work or in her personal life, before her depression began, she spent a lot of time becoming stressed about unimportant things. So, she gave up the obsession, hoping that this would allow her to heal from her depression.

Mary Anne enjoyed this time of not caring and not controlling everything. She felt relief for the first time in years. She set herself free and truly felt more liberated than ever.

When Mary Anne felt the fears and worries come to her mind again, she began to think of solutions. Now that her stress levels had decreased significantly, she had the energy to come up with some effective ways she can improve her life. She acknowledged that her depression changed her, but she knew she still had her good qualities—she still had many strengths, skills, and talents. Depression does not take that from you. Mary Anne knew this.

Mary Anne began to think of how she could use her strengths and positive qualities to pursue new goals and to fulfil her desire to get ahead in life. She still wanted to achieve many things, both personally and professionally. Depression did not take this from her either. This desire to live life and to achieve things is an important sign of progress for a person who has gone through depression

What allowed Mary Anne to get to this point was *acceptance*. It was when Mary Anne accepted herself and her state of depression and anxiety; when she accepted the outcomes in her life, she was able to see a possible, alternative path to her goals. This happened when she stopped fighting *against* herself and her emotions, and when she stopped judging herself for being depressed and anxious. She stopped caring, but what really happened was that she gave herself space to feel depressed.

The worrying, the self-criticism and the depression didn't allow Mary Anne to recover. All she saw was negativity and more and more problems. She finally surrendered to everything, to her depression, her excessively high expectations of herself, her need for perfection, her worries...*everything*. Mary Anne didn't realise it then, but she set herself free by discovering the power of acceptance.

Once Mary Anne stopped punishing herself, she was able to see all the options she had that she could use to improve her life; she saw the strengths and positive traits she still had in her, to pursue her goals.

Years later, Mary Anne shared with me that she was grateful for having gone through depression! Yes, she felt a sense of gratitude for that difficult time in her life. Acceptance also taught Mary Anne to have no regrets in her life. She only sees lessons. She only sees how everything that happened to her had a purpose.

Mary Anne looks back at her life now and only tells about the amazing journey she was fortunate enough to experience. Mary Anne still experiences hardship and struggles at times. She has both good days and bad days, but there is a difference now that she went through and recovered from depression.

Mary Anne does not see problems as the end of something. She sees challenges and hardships in life as a sign that something better is to come. She understands how life unfolds.

*We are brave, strong, and courageous because we were once afraid, weak, alone, and depressed.*

# Chapter TWELVE

# ASSERTIVENESS: THE DEPRESSION & ANXIETY REMEDY

I know this is a bold statement—to say that assertiveness can be a remedy for depression and anxiety. However, I have observed this to be true for far too long to ignore the very clear relationship between assertiveness and emotional health. Being assertive certainly doesn't solve everything when it comes to depression and anxiety, but it has a central role in how you see yourself and those you interact with.

Let's consider for a moment how non-assertive behaviour can contribute to depression or anxiety and how this specifically impacts you as a woman.

The culture you were raised in will influence your personality, the way you think, act, and behave, your values, and even your emotional health.

There are vast differences across cultures when it comes to the roles and behaviours of women, but I also believe there are stereotypes or characteristics expected of women that are, in my opinion, fairly cross-cultural, too. Assertiveness is one of those characteristics.

I think it's fair to say that in many cultures, women are socialised to be less assertive and quieter, reserved, more submissive, or overall, less assertive compared to men.

There are cultures where assertiveness is more encouraged or promoted among women, especially in this day and age; however, in general, men still tend to be more socialised to act in a more self-assured manner, show more confidence and strength, and overall to speak up and say what they want more than women. I also believe women are in the midst of a time where these types of differences between men and women are changing, and I am hopeful I will live to see the day both men and women are praised and supported equally for assertiveness. However, for the time being, non-assertive behaviour continues to be an area of struggle for many women.

Non-assertive behaviour certainly varies depending on the person. Some women may be far more assertive than others, while some may struggle more in some areas of life. For example, some women may be less assertive in their work/professional relationships. Sometimes, it's easier for some women to be more assertive with close loved ones or people they know well, as they may feel greater confidence that these people will love and accept them. Non-assertive behaviour can come from a belief or a fear that we will not be *accepted* or that we'll be *rejected* by others. Non-assertive behaviour is, therefore, a form of being submissive in order to avoid rejection or being criticised by others.

It is important to identify your own difficulties with being assertive. Being aware of the specific areas where you struggle is an important first step in increasing your assertiveness. Below are some examples of non-assertive behaviours, actions, and thought processes.

- Non-assertive people are usually less verbal, meaning they may want something or wish to say something to someone else, but often hold back from saying what they desire or need.
- If unhappy or dissatisfied with a situation, rather than saying so to the person or people involved, non-assertive people will usually stay silent and keep those feelings to themselves.
- It may seem like nothing bothers or upsets a non-assertive person because they don't often express disagreement. However, sometimes the opposite is true and they become very upset or emotional, but won't express how they feel.
- -Non-assertive people may avoid speaking up because they fear social rejection or social disapproval.
- They may feel that disagreeing will mean others will not like them or approve of them.

- Non-assertive people may fear hurting or disappointing others. They also happen to be highly sensitive individuals who would rather keep their feelings and desires to themselves instead of hurting or disappointing another person.
- Non-assertive people may be socially anxious. Social anxiety—a fear of speaking in front of others or of being embarrassed, rejected, or evaluated by others—is associated with a lack of assertiveness. A socially anxious person often fears making a mistake in front of others, looking unintelligent, or sounding/appearing "dumb"; therefore, they may not speak up or defend themselves to avoid humiliation.

You might recognise yourself in some or possibly all of these descriptions of a non-assertive person. If this is the case, try not to be hard on yourself for it and keep in mind that *all* people struggle with some incidences of non-assertiveness.

I believe, however, that building and developing your assertiveness is critical if you struggle with depression and anxiety. You see, as a woman with depression and anxiety, you're struggling with thoughts and feelings about yourself that are usually very negative. You might believe that your problems are too much for you to handle. Maybe you feel incapable of confronting life's greatest challenges. Does this sound like you?

In your interactions with others, you probably feel everyone else is greater, smarter, more talented, and more competent. You might step aside for other people or maybe you feel you're not deserving of good things and your needs are not important. The problem with all this is that if you don't see your needs as important, and if you can't speak openly and express your needs, you will likely end up missing out on what makes you happy.

Rejection is something you fear because when you are not accepted by others, you risk being abandoned and alone, two of the greatest fears of a non-assertive person. You greatly fear being alone because you believe you cannot make it or survive on your own. Do you see the underlying thoughts and feelings here?

So, in exchange for avoiding that loneliness you fear you make sure that you're socially accepted, whether it's by your spouse, family, children, other loved ones, friends, co-workers, or bosses. You will keep your thoughts, feelings, and ideas to yourself even if you're being treated wrongly or unfairly.

You are taking a great risk here, however, because your non-assertion and fear of loneliness expose you to potential mistreatment or even abuse. You do not value yourself; therefore, will others see your value and treat you with respect?

For many women, non-assertiveness turns into depression and anxiety because you keep your thoughts and feelings in. You don't express yourself when you need to. Particularly in relationships, this becomes problematic and can lead to various types of conflict. With time, your stress levels will increase.

As an assertive woman, you don't have to be available to others all the time. You know that you don't need to be complacent and agreeable to be loved and accepted. The reality is that to be truly loved and accepted by others, it is important to be genuine in your relationships, especially in close relationships. The popular term for this is "being yourself." Assertiveness is about speaking up for yourself, saying what you feel, and standing up for your needs. This is not selfishness. It is loving, valuing, and respecting yourself.An assertive woman is not unkind or unfair, although she may be accused of possessing these qualities by a society, a partner, loved ones, family members, or an employer who wishes to keep her subservient. Assertiveness means having enough respect and love for yourself, confidence in yourself, and being fine on your own if you must be, even if you're afraid.

That's another quality of the assertive woman: She *is* afraid like anyone else. An assertive women can feel fear of rejection, criticism, or isolation, but doesn't let that fear dictate how she will allow other people to treat her. The assertive woman doesn't allow fear to stop her from standing up for her rights, her needs, and her desires.

Assertiveness helps you set boundaries. It allows good people into your life and eliminates negative people and negative relationships.

Assertiveness will prevent others from taking advantage of you. It allows you to value yourself and your contribution to a relationship. Assertiveness allows you to enjoy relationships that are equal, where both you and the other person both contribute.So, all this talk about assertiveness leaves a very important question pending. How do you develop and increase your assertiveness, especially if, after reading this chapter, you realise you could benefit from practising some assertiveness skills?

Practising assertiveness involves developing a habit of speaking up for yourself and putting across your point of view in your day-to-day interactions. There are so many opportunities to practice it with others, you just have to keep it in mind so that you can speak up, verbalize, and express yourself instead of holding your thoughts and feelings *in*. Any time you feel the urge to *hold back*, you speak up instead.

I am not for a moment suggesting you become argumentative, abrasive, or generally hard to get along with! There is a difference. Simply ensure your voice is heard and that you express your wants and needs. That doesn't involve raising your voice, name-calling, shows of petulance or any other form of out-of-control behaviour. Assertive people are often also highly amiable and are great allies and friends. They are popular—in part because they carry themselves with confidence and stand up for their views and beliefs. Some people are "quietly confident." That means they have self-belief and assertiveness, but are quiet and reflective, too. The assertiveness trait does not mean you have to be dominant, loud, the centre of attention, controlling or domineering. Being assertive also does not mean that you will always get what you want in life, but this is not the point of being assertive anyways. Assertiveness is a release of thoughts and emotion. Releasing thoughts and emotions is healthier than keeping them within you where they can cause damage to your mental health and wellbeing.Like any other issue in self-improvement, the first step is admitting you have a problem with assertiveness. You might be surprised to know that many women I've talked to about assertiveness through the years will think of many excuses to explain their lack of assertiveness. Ironically, they hold up their argument with much assertiveness—yet in most other areas, they retreat from putting forth their needs! I think the true reason for women having difficulty admitting to this problem goes back to fear, but in this case, the fear of change.

Think about it this way; if they admitted to lacking assertiveness, this would put them in a position where change would be warranted, and they'd have to finally do something about their lack of assertiveness.

After you take an honest look at the circumstances in your own life; at your stressors; your relationships; and the factors contributing to your depression and anxiety, you can then identify where you could benefit from being more assertive. It could be an issue in practically every area of your life or isolated to one or two areas, such as work-life or romantic relationships.

Once you have identified this area of need, you can begin to practice.

Yes, since assertiveness is partly a habit, improving it will involve practice. This practice involves giving your thoughts and feelings a voice, so instead of keeping thoughts and feelings to yourself, you will begin to speak them in situations where you have historically held back. Ask yourself in such situations: What do *I* want? Do the people in the room/in my life know this is what I want? Can I make it evident to them?

Many women have also shared with me that they worry about no longer being kind, caring, and giving when they begin to stand up for themselves and their needs. It might seem this way at first, but with practice, you will learn to see the beauty in the balance of asserting yourself while also maintaining kindness and consideration of others.

Now, bear in mind this exercise will likely lead to some adversity from others when you start to speak up, but this will be a signal that your assertiveness is finally shining through. And those who truly respect and care for you will commend you for committing to be more assertive if it means that you are working towards greater happiness, self-value, and self-esteem. You can even do this with much humour by telling loved ones you're going to try being more assertive and that they can help you along the way by pointing out when you're not standing up for your needs. Have a laugh about it, too.

Humour defuses any sense of abrasiveness others may feel at seeing the new you.

Know, too, that learning to be assertive can be uncomfortable at first. You might even find yourself blushing or developing a slight stammer, or some other overt sign of unease. Again, you can laugh it off or simply say nothing. It's unlikely anyone will notice it and if they do, so what?

Believe me, almost everyone is way too busy and preoccupied worrying about how they come across to others, to notice or be concerned about you.

This is a useful realisation to understand. Recognise that pretty much everyone around you also has some degree of insecurity or vulnerability. When you think everyone's staring at you and picking out all your inadequacies—they're really not. They're lost in their own worries about how everyone else—including you—sees *them*.

# *Chapter* THIRTEEN

# COPING WITH LOSS & DEVELOPING RESILIENCE

Loss can come to your life suddenly and unexpectedly. The story of Lilly reminds me of how even those who seem to have the most perfect and ideal life can receive a very harsh lesson in loss.

Lilly struggled with a very difficult loss, but still kept an outer appearance of happiness, as if her life was pure bliss at all times. She wasn't arrogant about her life of privilege, but always appeared unbothered and relaxed. Lilly had a nice home and three polite young children.

She had a devoted husband. They all had dinner together every night, did family activities together on weekends, and Lilly and her husband even went out alone together one night every week. Lilly's husband was an overall "nice guy," and Lilly was madly in love with him.

The feeling was seemingly mutual, as he appeared as if his whole world revolved around Lilly and the children. Could her life be any more perfect?

Well, Lilly's life journey took a sudden and drastic turn one day when she used her husband's laptop to buy film tickets for the children. His browser was open to his email account. Lilly coincidentally saw a suspicious subject line in one of the e-mails and... everything changed for Lilly from that moment forward. There was a long trail of e-mails revealing, in detail, her husband's infidelity.

Lilly was shocked and horrified. I would say the whole experience was a real trauma, as Lilly discussed and repeated to me how she and her husband had not been having any marital issues—or, at least, as far as she was aware—that could explain her husband's infidelity. Lilly was overcome with feelings of grief, deep loss, and utter shock.

Hearing Lilly tell me this story was heart breaking. Several times, I almost felt like asking her to stop describing the terrible things she discovered about her husband, but as I saw the tears streaming down her face and heard the despair and anger in her trembling voice, I couldn't be so selfish as to ask her to spare me the details.

Lilly did what many women do, but often don't admit to: She forgave her husband. When she confronted him about the emails to *more than three women* (her husband had had at least three affairs within a span of approximately five years) he told her he was still in love with her and those relationships meant nothing to him. Lilly achieved some peace when her husband confessed to being unfaithful, but him begging her not to leave him and reassuring her he was still in love with her made it difficult for Lilly to make a decision about the possibility of leaving him and moving on with her life.

With time, and after forgiving her husband, Lilly didn't seem able to move on fully. She was experiencing a lot of physical ailments that had no medical explanation after seeing her doctor. She suffered from headaches, stomach aches, and had difficulty sleeping from time to time.

One day, in one of my meetings with Lilly, she asked me for advice on how to handle her present situation. She had asked for advice before, but I had always been hesitant to specifically tell her what I thought she should do. I felt the incident was too recent, and I didn't want to influence her decision-making. I felt Lilly needed to make this big decision for herself. However, one day, she looked me in the eye and asked me directly what my thoughts were about her situation.

I thought for a moment and then responded with what I would want or wish for a friend to advise me if I were in Lilly's situation. I told her that I felt that she needed time to breathe, to think, to be alone with herself. I feel that to cope with loss and deal with betrayal, Lilly had to take some time to be alone with herself so that she could think and evaluate what was best for her.

You see, Lilly, as a dedicated wife and mother, always put herself second. To a certain extent, it's understandable that a mother will make her children and family a priority, even above her own needs and desires; however, Lilly was fully immersed in the identities of wife and mother.This loss of identity prevented her from being able to decide what she truly wanted in her life and what would make her happy. However, after her husband's infidelity—and as time passed—Lilly realised she had to be truly happy so that she could be a good mother, wife, or *person*.Lilly knew she was unhappy in her marriage because, after several months, she was unable to recover from her husband's infidelity. She tried to continue with her marriage. Lilly knew that if she was going to forgive her husband, she would have to "forget" everything that happened. Lilly was unable to do this, which is why I—and she—believed she was struggling with so many physical complaints and health concerns. It is common for the body to express a lot of what the mind can't handle.

Lilly and I talked about her life and her future. She acknowledged she still had many years of life to live. She considered whether she was being fair to herself, her children, and even to her husband if she were to live out the remaining years of her life in an unhappy state. Looking at her situation in this way helped Lilly make decisions. For a long time after discovering her husband's infidelity, she had been thinking mostly short-term and ignoring the fact that she knew she could not remain unhappy for the rest of her life.

Lilly and I discussed how her being unhappy and struggling with health issues could destroy her lively and positive spirit, possibly turning her into a bitter and resentful person. How would this impact the way her children saw her? They were young and needed her, and she knew she could not hide her feelings from them. Children are extremely intuitive and can feel when one or both parents are having emotional issues.

You might be able to guess what happened at the end of Lilly's story. It was actually the beginning of her story.Well, Lilly ultimately filed for divorce from her husband exactly fourteen months after she learned of his infidelity. Among the many things Lilly realized, she was certain she was no longer able to trust him fully. Lilly is a very genuine person and felt she was living a lie. She also found that a divorce did not mean that her family was broken. Instead, Lilly felt she made her family whole again when she made a decision that was right for her. She felt she was only giving her children half of the mother they deserved because she was so unfulfilled and unhappy.

The divorce was amicable, and Lilly is so much happier now. She took her loss and used it to find herself again.

# Chapter FOURTEEN

# ENHANCE YOUR WELL-BEING THROUGH SELF-TALK

I *strongly* believe that it is only through self-love, self-compassion, and forgiving yourself that you can truly heal. Your self-talk is very important in your ability to achieve love, compassion, forgiveness, and healing.

## THE RELATIONSHIP BETWEEN SELF-TALK AND BEING KIND TO YOURSELF

Women often learn to be strict, critical, and harsh with themselves because they believe they *must* be this way to improve, succeed, and progress in life.

The reality is that the gentler you are on yourself and the more self-forgiving you are, the greater the likelihood you'll be able to heal from or cope with emotional struggles and get through life's greatest difficulties. Being gentle with yourself is especially important when those around you may not be as kind towards you as you need. If you know you can rely on yourself as your primary source of emotional support, the occasional conflicts in your relationships with others will not impact you so severely.

There is a direct relationship between your internal dialogues, also known as your *self-talk*, and how you feel, how you behave, and how you see the world around you. *Your internal dialogue is also related to the kindness and compassion you show yourself.*

## WHEN THEY TELL YOU: "IT'S ALL IN YOUR MIND"

Most women know how it feels when family members, friends, a spouse or partner, or co-workers give unhelpful "advice" on how you should deal with your depression. Although others may have good intentions, those who have never struggled with depression may believe that depression is something you have control over—something you can "turn off" by "not thinking about it" or "thinking positive thoughts." Sadly, loved ones might even insist that your depression is *all in your mind*, implying that it isn't *real*. When those you love and trust do not validate your feelings, you might feel very lonely, sad, and frustrated.Plus, when you're struggling to cope with emotions, the last thing you want to hear is someone offering you unrealistic "advice." If it were so easy to eliminate depression, you would have certainly done it by now. Alleviating depression—and eventually recovering from it—involves a process of learning and personal growth. Positive thinking *is* part of this process, but there is a specific method of really making positive thinking a part of your life.

## POSITIVE THINKING: IT ACTUALLY DOES WORK

I will do my best to explain these ideas in this chapter, but what I won't tell you is that it's all going to be easy for you. It's not easy. It will take you much training and practice because you must retrain your brain to *think* and perceive things differently, which is not a simple task, especially if you tend to be very strict, critical, and harsh with yourself.Keep in mind these two primary principles:

1. Your thoughts and beliefs, including the "messages" you say to yourself, also known as your internal dialogue, influence how you act or behave *and* how you feel emotionally.
2. How you interpret or comprehend events and things that happen to you in your life also influences how you act or behave *and* how you feel emotionally.

Although these two points might be easy to understand, making the changes in your life might take some time.

I have found a good place to start is by understanding that—as I mentioned earlier in the book—*you are not your thoughts*.

*What?*

This is a confusing concept for some people. If you are familiar with mindfulness, then you might understand this well. If not, spend some time thinking about it as we discuss this more in this chapter.

You are not your thoughts is one of the greatest truths I've discovered in my life that I would like to share with you.

## SEPARATING THE SELF (YOU) FROM THOUGHT

It is a strange idea—that you are not your thoughts—because your thoughts, your *mind*, is what navigates the world for you. It is what helps you understand, interact, feel, think, remember, see, and listen. Your mind is the control centre of your identity, but this is also precisely why you must ignore your mind—or the thought that your mind comes up with—most of the time. Thoughts help you work, interact with people, get things accomplished, etcetera, but aside from using your mind for these practical purposes, you shouldn't pay attention to it or believe many of the thoughts your mind develops.

Basically, I am saying that you would be better off ignoring your mind. But, is this possible? You see, your mind works like a reflex. The mind can work in a very primitive manner. Think of the knee-jerk reflex. This is a lot like how your mind works. This is also why your thoughts can be negative, unrealistic, or completely crazy.

I'll give you a good example.

Did you know many people often report that when they go to the bank and approach the teller to complete a transaction, they have the most unusual thought when they see stacks and stacks of cash behind the teller desk? They fantasise about what it would be like to rob the bank and be able to take all that money with them! Of course, most people realise their thought is completely unrealistic because the majority of customers would never rob a bank. However, there is something about seeing that amount of money that makes many people think: *What if I took it all?*

The thought is merely a reaction to seeing piles of money at the teller desk, money that you know takes a lot of time and hard work to make. How nice would it be to be able to take a mere handful of that cash. Imagine if people internalised these thoughts and believed them true. Imagine if the person thinking this began to believe they must be a thief. Surely, if they thought of robbing the bank and taking the cash from the teller, they *must* be a criminal.

Having these thoughts does not mean the person would rob the bank, harm other people, and commit a serious crime. They realise their mind produced a silly thought, and it makes them smile for a moment. The majority of people dismiss those thoughts immediately.

This example provides another two important pieces of information to keep in mind when considering why you must separate yourself from your mind or thoughts.

1. Your mind will produce all sorts of *crazy* thoughts and ideas, like a knee-jerk reflex, on a constant basis.
2. Those thoughts and ideas *do not* represent or define who you are.

Keeping these three points in mind is especially important when struggling with depression or anxiety because you will invariably experience negative and self-defeating thoughts and beliefs. Depression and anxiety develop and get worse when you believe *you are* those thoughts and beliefs, and those thoughts and beliefs are you.

However, if you can grasp how you and your thoughts are separate entities, you'll gradually, but surely, distance yourself from the sadness, the fear, the worry, the self-doubt, and the numerous other thoughts and emotions that result from negative thoughts and beliefs.

What comes out of this separation of self and thought/mind is magical. Some people even call it true freedom! When you detach from reacting to your thoughts, when you truly understand that you should not "believe" what your thoughts "say" to you, then depression and anxiety can diminish. For many people, depression and anxiety can even *disappear* when you no longer identify with your thoughts. Just as the bank customer doesn't believe she's a thief—that she would rob the bank and steal the cash—you shouldn't believe the irrational, sad, unrealistic, or negative thoughts that pass through your mind.

As with any new skill or ability, it takes practice to master it. The process is not difficult, and all you need is quite a bit of persistence. As you practice, you will begin to see the benefits. You will begin to see your thoughts for what they are, *just thoughts*.

A great exercise for beginners is the observation exercise where you spend some time—maybe weeks, maybe months—becoming *the watcher* or *observer* of your thoughts. Observe where your thoughts wander off to throughout the day and what they try to tell you. Observe how your mind works like a reflex, making irrational conclusions all the time. Observe how your thoughts can be negative, "telling you" things that put you down or make you feel badly about yourself.

Your thoughts will even try hard to convince you when you try to resist them. Once you become aware of your thoughts—once you can put yourself in the place of watcher and observer—you have already made a huge accomplishment. You have already created the self-thought separation.

Consider the following example about how powerful and convincing thoughts can be.

## THE STORY OF WENDY

Wendy just joined a local book club, and she's attending the very first club meeting. She's a new member, but she's aware some women who will be present are long-time members who have belonged to the club for years. On the day of the

> first book club meeting, Wendy walks into the meeting room, which is a large auditorium with other activities taking place.
>
> She sees the table where the club members agreed to meet, and it looks like a few of the members have already sat down at the table. Wendy approaches, a bit nervous about meeting strangers, but excited to make some new friends.
>
> As she gets close to an empty chair at the table, Wendy looks around at the four other women already seated. She smiles at them and says hello. Then, there's a long pause as Wendy waits for someone to acknowledge her greeting, but all she can hear is the distant voices of other people in the auditorium.
>
> Wendy awkwardly sits down, takes her book out of her purse. She looks down at the pages, although she's not reading anything. All Wendy keeps *thinking* is how embarrassed she feels that all the women *ignored* her. *Nobody likes her. She shouldn't have bothered coming.* Her mind keeps working and her thoughts turn more and more negative.
>
> Not knowing what to do, Wendy sits for a minute, but then suddenly gets up, leaves the auditorium, and decides not to continue attending meetings.

Wendy's reaction at the book club might seem abrupt, but this true story is an excellent example of the way the mind can make decisions, conclusions, and create so many thoughts that can be completely untrue. Why would Wendy forget about how excited she'd been to join the book club and decide to quit just because no one greeted her at the table? She quit because she believed all those thoughts about *why* no one greeted her.

You see, Wendy is a very kind person who enjoyed socialising, but she tended to be a bit shy around strangers. Once she felt comfortable with a new friend or group, she was able to relax and enjoy the interaction; however, she always struggled with meeting new people and joining groups due to a fear of rejection and a deep desire to be liked and accepted. Wendy tended to have doubts about whether people would like her, as she believed they would think she was dull, boring, and not outgoing or social enough. Well, when Wendy approached the table at the book club meeting and did not receive a greeting in return, she was immediately overwhelmed with those negative thoughts and beliefs about herself.

As she sat at the table, looking down at her book, her mind "told her" that the book club members must not want her there, that they may not like the way she looked, or that maybe they noticed her strange accent when she said hello. Wendy believed her mind—her thoughts—so she never returned to the club.

Now, let's look at things differently. Let's say Wendy turned into the watcher or the observer of her thoughts. What would have been different for her in this situation? Maybe Wendy can notice the negative thoughts, observe them as if she was watching a film or TV show, and then, without judging herself, allow those thoughts to pass her by. Wendy can acknowledge that those thoughts are a product of some of the things she struggles with, mainly her self-esteem, but she can also acknowledge those thoughts are separate from her, the person *she* really is.

Wendy's thoughts are a reflex reaction. Many of the negative beliefs she has about herself started long ago when she was rejected by peers in school and years later, by her ex-fiancé, by her co-workers, and even by her older sister. However, now, Wendy can *observe* her thoughts.

She can see it as an onlooker instead of a participant.

Wendy doesn't need to identify with those thoughts as if they were true or real. Those thoughts are *not* who she is. She is the observer now, watching the thoughts as they come to her mind and then imagining them *move past her*.

When Wendy becomes the observer, her thoughts no longer control her and take hold of her. She is in control of herself, and the thoughts no longer dictate her feelings and actions. The thoughts no longer make Wendy feel hurt by what she "thinks" is rejection. Her thoughts no longer cause her to get up and leave the table. She no longer believes the emotions of humiliation or embarrassment are her emotions. She no longer "owns" those emotions. She acknowledges that the thoughts are merely habitual reactions repeating themselves each time Wendy finds herself in a social situation.

Wendy now knows there are many possibilities for why the women did not respond when she said hello. It's possible that since the room was too busy with noise and activity, the ladies seated at the table they did not hear Wendy's greeting. She also knows they might have seen her arrive at the table, but assumed she was greeting someone else. Maybe the ladies realized Wendy was saying hello, but recognised it too late and Wendy had already turned to look down at her book when they smiled and greeted her back. It's also very possible that the ladies at the table were feeling insecure in the social setting, too, just like Wendy. They were lost in their own thoughts and maybe didn't hear Wendy's greeting! There are so many possibilities that could explain why Wendy didn't receive a greeting in return. However, if you struggle with depression, your mind may tend to develop negative thoughts, responses, and "explanations" for events and situations in your environment.

Thoughts can create a "story" about how everyone is judging you even when the reverse could be true.

Remind yourself of the following truth: *These are thoughts, but I don't have to listen to them.*

Chapter

FIFTEEN

# DEVELOPING SELF-LOVE & SEEKING HEALTHY LOVE

When was the last time you asked yourself:

*"How much do I love myself?"*

There is connection between your level of self-love and:

- ❖ Your self-esteem
- ❖ Your ability to be more compassionate towards yourself
- ❖ Your ability to forgive yourself for past mistakes, let go of the past, and move on.

Self-love is also very much related to the quality of your relationships, whether you let toxic people into your life, and whether or not you know when to move past relationships that are unhealthy for you.

Self-love helps you set boundaries and show assertiveness. It gives you the confidence to say "no" when you need to. Self-love contributes to happiness, well-being, and a better quality of life. When you are confronted with life stressors and challenges, self-love can help you cope.

Self-love is critical because *you have to love yourself before you can love anyone else*; before you can truly enjoy relationships.

You also have to *love yourself before you can expect anyone else to love you.*

*Fall in love with yourself, so you don't have to look for someone else to fill that need.*

If you don't have a good source of self-love, you may look for love outside of yourself, in your relationships with others. Although it is perfectly fine and *human* to want love from others, your source of love for yourself must also exist. This is what makes you able to fully enjoy love from others and prevent having relationships based on unhealthy dependency. It is not arrogance to have self-love, but a healthy regard for the self.

We often do not learn about the importance of self-love. Women especially are raised to be nurturing of others—to put the needs of others before their own—and this is seen as being an admirable quality. Although it *is* admirable to be selfless, this teaching is missing a huge component not emphasized nearly as much as it should be, and that is *self-love*. If you want to nurture and care for others without expecting anything in return, and if you want to fulfil the needs of those you love and at times, even put the needs of others before your own, you're going to need self-love. Self-love gives you balance and strength to be able to be there for others when they need you.

## SELF-LOVE AND TOXIC RELATIONSHIPS

Self-love also helps you to distinguish between people who *only* "take" in relationships rather than "give and take." Self-love helps you to set boundaries with these types of people that may come into your life.

Self-love also helps you to seek out healthy relationships and people you deserve, not people who wish to take advantage of you.

Surrounding yourself with people who are capable of sharing in an empathic relationship with you is critical. If you currently have toxic people in your life or have let these people into your life in the past, don't blame yourself or question your judgment. I believe highly empathic people often go through a series of toxic relationships because empaths attract people in need of a lot of healing. In achieving greater self-love, you will be able to learn to identify these people and these types of toxic relationships so you can avoid them in future.

Your growing self-love will also help you to understand that it's not your job to heal other people, particularly toxic ones affecting you negatively. You can show these people where they can seek resources to get help, but it's not up to you to sacrifice your well-being for the sake of trying to help a toxic person or mend a damaging relationship with someone else.

A big part of a personal test of self-love will be your ability to let these people/relationships go and find peace in doing so.

# Chapter SIXTEEN

# FINDING MEANING: HOW YOU CAN USE WHAT YOU HAVE LEARNED TO HELP OTHERS

Below is a story as told by Hannah, a single mother who suffers from depression. Hannah does not let her depression rule her life. She has learned that a strategy that helps her cope is helping those around her. This brings much meaning to Hannah's life, as well as a sense of purpose for the struggles she has experienced due to depression.

*I've had a very challenging day today because I've experienced a lot of depression. I've experienced a lot of feelings of loneliness, separation, frustration, anger, hurt, and I have had a victim mindset. I am not sure how many times I've cried today. And yet, I think I've helped more people today, than on most of my good days.*

*I go to Alcoholics Anonymous (AA)—as I am an alcoholic—daily, and what I like about AA is that it's a place where I can honestly share how my day is going. I don't have to show up, look good and try to impress people and say, "Well, yes, I'm having a great day," when in fact, I'm not.*

*But there are lots of other places I can go to get help, apart from therapy meetings. I can get support from a family member or friend, from people at work, or wherever I feel I can honestly and safely share my feelings without getting condemned or judged.*

*And I'm finding that the people who supported me the most are often the ones who are in the middle of a bad day themselves. They then, in turn, talk about what they're feeling; thus, they are confiding in me as much as I am confiding in them. And the reason I think it's so helpful is that when you hear that on a good day, then it brings gratitude.*

*I probably wouldn't have made it this far in my life without so many loving people showing me unconditional acceptance and just letting me share what I'm feeling.*

*It is society's norm that, as a woman, you always need to look good and feel good to fit in. You need to look good all day, every day, go to work, take care of the kids, be there for your husband, and you then come home and not have any problems. A lot of us have been programmed to focus on looking good all the time.*

*And, you know what? I don't look good today. I've been crying. That is how my days appear. And that's real. That's the inside of my life.*

*But it does not stop there. These days are great days to help other people learn things and make progress.*

Everyone deals depression in different ways. Some try to handle it by themselves while others get help and talk about their feelings, like Hannah. Support from others is an excellent way to cope. Having the ability to be your own source of support is critical, but this does not take away the importance of seeking support from others.

There are also certain methods you can do for yourself that could help. It is best to achieve a balance where you seek support from others while also develop your ability to support yourself through depression. Below are a few other self-care ideas you might want to try.

## JOURNALING

Research has examined how journaling can help to alleviate and prevent depression, and the results are very promising. Journaling forces you to express yourself and reflect on your thoughts and feelings. If you're not accustomed to journaling, it might seem strange, but give it a try! You might be amazed at the emotional release journaling can give you. It also helps greatly to write down your thoughts and feelings so you can refer to what you wrote later on. This allows you to challenge and replace negative thoughts and beliefs with more positive alternatives.

## RECONNECTING WITH A FRIEND

Even if you have no desire to get out and talk to people (this is common in depression), it can be very helpful to make a small effort to increase your exposure to social situations, even if only for a short period of time on a weekly basis. Researchers have looked at the most effective strategies for dealing with depression, and actively participating in your own social life is very beneficial. Humans are social beings, so we benefit from being a part of a community. This does not mean that you can't spend time alone. In fact, it is also healthy to dedicate time to yourself and enjoy this time. However, time spent on social connection is also important.

Depression can make you feel like doing just about anything is an extreme effort, especially going out anywhere. However, what is important here is to avoid being too ambitious. You don't need to plan long and complicated social outings. Even just exposing yourself for 15 minutes in a public setting, and then building up from that point, is enough to ensure that you maintain social contact.

## COMFORT FOOD

Certain foods and diet have a strong effect on depression. You could challenge yourself to maintain a very healthy diet, as this can improve your overall mood. There are certain foods that have antidepressant qualities, including chocolate, tea, and coffee. It is typically best to avoid foods that contain processed sugar, as well as high carbohydrate foods, as consuming foods from both of these categories can cause sudden increases in your blood sugar followed by a sudden decrease in blood sugar. This can significantly lead to low energy and rapid shifts in how you feel both physically and emotionally.

## HUMOUR

You've all heard that saying, *laughter is the best medicine* and it is very true! Humour is a great way to cope with depression. Watch a funny movie, see a stand-up comedian; do whatever makes you laugh. Laughter releases endorphins and decreases stress hormones, among many other benefits.

## PHYSICAL ACTIVITY

Sometimes, the simplest solutions are the most effective. Research has shown that regular, vigorous exercise is one of the best ways to fight depression. Exercise releases endorphins, which are natural feel-good chemicals in the body. The physical changes in our body that occur due to regular exercise is also excellent for self-esteem. How you feel about your appearance will not lead to a healthy self-esteem if you don't like your inner self, but liking how you look physically is *part* of *maintaining* a healthy self-esteem.

You might not be *eager* to exercise when you're depressed, so aim for only 10 minutes of exercise on those days when you're energy and motivation are low. After just 10 minutes, your mood and energy levels can increase significantly!

## VIDEO THERAPY

Another method of dealing with depression is video therapy. Although the word might sound complicated, it's pretty simple, and it's probably one of the most popular self-guided forms of therapy out there. Usually, there's an initial consultation with a professional therapist, and then the patient uses book readings to guide oneself along the therapy journey. The book instructs the client on various ways to cope with depression and conquer anxiety. One thing to keep in mind is that it's only recommended for those with mild depressive symptoms.

## YOGA

Some say yoga is just another form of exercise, but the truth is that it's so much more than a good way to build endurance and lean muscle. Many people describe yoga as a kind of meditation in motion; it can be spiritual, and also very introspective. It's certainly the case that yoga's meditation component is a large part of what makes it effective for depression. Yoga allows the mind to be still and the very fact that it requires concentration on postures is effective in drawing the mind to the present moment, resulting in greater mental clarity.

Meditation might be one of the oldest self-care techniques in history, since people have been meditating for thousands of years, and the effects of this practice are well documented. The goal of meditation is to attain inner peace, making it a perfect strategy for combating depression. One of the most popular methods for dealing with depression these days is mindfulness, which is a type of meditation.

## MASSAGE THERAPY

It's always good to treat yourself to a nice massage even when you have no specific mental health issues. But if you're trying to pursue a lifestyle of self-care, you might also want to consider massage therapy, as there are many benefits.

Massage therapy can assist a depressed person in decreasing stress levels and bringing a generalised sense of warmth and wellness to the body, as well as lifting the spirits. It is a temporary form of physical and mental relief, but with regular use, it can have more lasting effects.

# Chapter SEVENTEEN

# HOW YOUR MOOD IMPACTS DEPRESSION

Low mood and depression are really common and go hand in hand. Between one in four and one in five people experiences a significant low mood at some time in their life. So, you're definitely not alone! Sometimes the symptoms are short term, and may improve within a few weeks without you having to get treatment. But at other times, you can feel down and stop enjoying things for many weeks, months, or even longer.

When you get stuck in a period of low mood or depression, it can affect different aspects of your life. It can be hard to know what to do to improve the way you feel. Perhaps you can't sleep, or you tired and lethargic, or your self-confidence is gone. You feel stressed out, have a decreased appetite and feel like pushing people away.

These are just some of the ways low mood can affect you.

If you feel like you need help with breaking out of this cycle, the great news is there are so many treatment options available, such as Cognitive Behavioural Therapy (CBT), which is a popular and evidence-based form of talking therapy. CBT is developed to help you understand how your thoughts, feelings, and behaviour connect to keep you from feeling bad. CBT is best delivered in therapy, but if therapy isn't accessible to you, there are many excellent resources online that can help you learn some of the principles yourself. Podcasts and YouTube videos are accessible to anyone and provide so much information about CBT, as well as many more strategies to help combat your depression. Even if you're not yet ready to kick into action and address your depressive emotions and thoughts, simply listening to a good self-help podcast or video can boost your mood and increase your motivation.

People often think about depression as just being low in mood. But it's far more than that. It can affect every aspect of our lives.

Here's a typical example of Darlene experiencing and tackling low mood.

Darlene had a job she enjoyed, but when the recession hit she was laid off. She was left feeling more and more depressed as time passed. She tried to suppress her feelings, but eventually told her doctor about her symptoms. Her doctor was very helpful and drew a diagram to help Darlene understand how all those different symptoms fit together to create the thought-feeling-behaviour cycle that leads to depression and how this affects her feelings.

The doctor also asked Darlene how she was feeling in five key areas of her life. He was helping her think about the people and events around her and the impact of all this has on her thoughts, feelings, physical symptoms, and behaviour.

This so-called five area assessment is aimed at helping Darlene understand her situation better and to motivate her to make some small changes that can have a big impact on how she feels and her overall functioning.

The first of the five areas comprises the people and events around us. Let's use Darlene's situation to think through how this applies to her. Darlene has lots of things going on around her that cause her to feel much worry and pressure about her current situation and her future.

She has lost her job and feels she does not have enough money to get through the month and since losing her job, she has stopped seeing her friends as much as she used to. She feels she doesn't know anybody and therefore, feels isolated and lonely. There are other things too. One of her friends is very unwell, and she is having conflict with a neighbour.

These are just a few example of the sorts of stressors that can go wrong around you and can contribute to your depression getting worse. What Darlene didn't know before her chat with her doctor was that her life stress could cause a vicious circle making her feel worse inside. In addition, having depression makes it difficult to manage stress effectively; meaning that things that Darlene would normally be able to handle without a problem suddenly seem like a much bigger deal.

Let's move on to look at the second of the five areas. For the past three months, Darlene had been thinking and saying to herself, "Could I have done more or worked harder? What if I don't find a new job? I'm too embarrassed to tell my friends and family I've been laid off. I should not feel this way. I should be strong and confident."

All these unhelpful thoughts are common in depression and include self-critical things like "I'm hopeless, I have nothing to offer," or second-guessing yourself and worrying about what others think, such as "people think I'm useless."

Depression makes you blame yourself for things that aren't your fault. These are all unhelpful thoughts. They often aren't true, but depression causes you to dwell on these thoughts, almost like your brain gets stuck on anything and everything negative, making you feel worse.

This leads to the third area called altered feelings. Have you ever noticed that what you think can affect how you feel emotionally? Because Darlene's mind is so full of negative and self-critical thoughts, she feels worse emotionally. She feels down, guilty, fed up, angry, and stressed. She also notices one of the key symptoms in a low mood. Life stops feeling enjoyable, and that can affect her physically.

The physical aspect of depression is area four: altered physical feelings or sensations. People are often surprised at quite how physically exhausting low mood can be, and in this case, it leaves Darlene feeling physically exhausted. She also isn't feeling hungry anymore and has lost some weight. She is tired and feels run down, aches all over, and has headaches.

Other physical sensations that change during depression include feeling sick, palpitations, sweating and clamminess, going hot or cold, non-specific aches and pains, loss of sex drive, and a churning stomach. It is also important to know that depression and stress can lower the immune system quite dramatically, so associated viral infections also become common—and it is at this time when many people may first fall seriously ill on top of everything else they're going through! Immune disorders can be seriously debilitating and have long-term effects, but interestingly, many sufferers find these problems can self-resolve when the stress and depression lessen, over time. This shows the marked correlation between the mind and body; do not under-estimate it!

The altered thoughts, feelings and physical symptoms of the above list all add up to affect what Darlene does, having a knock-on effect on her behaviour and activity levels.

This brings us to the fifth and final area of the five areas assessment, which is the vicious cycle of depression whereby the worse Darlene feels, the less she does, and the less she does, the worse she feels. She stops looking for jobs and stays inside much of the day because she feels guilty about not being employed. As a result of this, she also stops visiting her family because she is embarrassed about having been laid off plus being around her family reminds her of how much of a failure she feels like.

When Darlene's sister calls her, Darlene shouts at her when her sister asks how things are going and if she has a new job yet. She has also stopped cooking meals, something that Darlene had a keen interest in and enjoyed doing before.

Finally, avoiding phone calls from her friends is cutting her off from another important possible source of support.

Other common health behaviours include drinking too much, over-sleeping, comfort eating, and putting important things off like paying bills or doing housework. All these—if you fall prey to them too—just worsen how you feel.

The good news is that this vicious circle spins both ways. By making a positive change in one area, things may change in other areas, too. Darlene and her doctor both agree her altered behaviour is a good place to start making changes.

As a small first step, Darlene decides to say yes to an invitation to go to her friends for Sunday lunch. She also decides she will start speaking to her friends and family on the phone again and listen to how they are doing rather than the conversation being focused on her.

She cooked herself a meal and found she enjoyed it. She does all these things bit by bit over the next few days. Thus, the activities are realistic, small and achievable. They're all things that will give her a renewed sense of pleasure and achievement, or closeness to others.

Darlene had a great day at the lunch with her friends then came home and chatted with her family to tell them about the outing.

Try working through your own five areas assessment and see if there are any changes you can make to help you feel better. Writing the process down is a good idea.

Firstly, think about what's going on in your life? Are there any pressures or problems present that are weighing you down?

Secondly, consider what's been going on in your mind recently? Are there any thoughts, memories or pictures or predictions you have about what will happen to you in the future?

Thirdly, from an emotional perspective, how does thinking about all of this make you feel? Low or maybe sad? Anxious, guilty, ashamed or angry?

Fourth, have you noticed you've been feeling different physically? If so, in what ways?

And finally, have you stopped doing things you used to enjoy? Are you avoiding anything? Or have you started doing new things that are becoming unhelpful or are contributing to you feeling sad? What impact has this altered activity had on how you're feeling?

Are you caught in a vicious circle?

If you feel you are, here's how to get out of it.

Firstly, watch out for upsetting thoughts that can affect how you feel emotionally and/or physically, or otherwise affect what you do. These are often just a thinking habit rather than being actual facts or truths. Sometimes just noticing the pattern will help you take a step back and change things.

Secondly, think of your physical symptoms. If you notice new symptoms that concern you, get them checked out by your doctor to find out if there is an underlying medical cause.

And if low mood or stress is worsening things, try anxiety control training and learn key coping skills to help relax your body and mind.

Thirdly, have a look at your behaviour. Getting going again is one of the best things you can do. Plan things that give you a sense of achievement, pleasure, and closeness to others, and make sure you re-establish a structure to your day by getting up and going to bed at a reasonable time. Eat three reasonable meals a day and say 'yes I can' rather than 'no I can't.' Negative thoughts tell you to say no and decline invitations. So, watch out for saying no to things before thinking whether it might be good if you push yourself just a bit and do it.

You're avoiding things because you feel scared, but the more you avoid things, the more it saps your confidence, and that vicious circle starts spinning again. Here are a few more don'ts: Don't drink too much or eat too much to block how you feel or push people away. Don't hide away or isolate yourself. Making changes can help boost your mood and help you feel better, which in turn will help you tackle whatever life throws at you.

So, go on, go for it and live your life to the fullest.

Chapter

EIGHTEEN

# HOW TO MANAGE ANXIETY WITH MINDFULNESS: A STEP-BY-STEP GUIDE

Managing anxiety and being able to switch off and relax a little each day can help you to stay well. Holidays and short dates can also make you feel great. But as you know, this can cost a lot in terms of time and money. Holidays also don't come around anywhere near often enough so we cannot rely on these moments in life to relax. We must implement other methods, too.

What I'm suggesting here is that you take a holiday every day, or even twice a day, but without the cost, the travel and the pain of lost bags, and all that spending. You need to learn a technique to help you relax and focus your mind away from worries and stress. Just sit back comfortably; let your gaze rest upon the point you've chosen.

And as the relaxation continues, your eyes may wish to close to enjoy a deeper calm, in which case they will.

Firstly, think about your hands. Think about the position of your hands, making slight contact or the pressure of the palms of your hands, the tips of your fingers and any feelings of warmth or coolness. Just being aware of the temperature of the skin of your hands and whether they're warm or cool will help as well. Notice any other feelings, perhaps a slight tingling feeling in your hands.

Now, think about the position of your arms and your shoulders resting back. Just being aware of any tension or tightness in the muscles of your arms around your shoulders and neck will help you centre your thoughts.

Notice that the tension or tightness is now replaced by relaxation. Your arms are now beginning to feel limp and relaxed. Let this controlled relaxation vibrate all through your body.

Next, concentrate on your feet and legs, just like your hands and arms. Take note of your feet and all the feelings you notice there, such as the position of your feet and the warmth or coolness. Just be aware of the temperature of the skin of your feet, whether they're warm, or cool, and other feelings. Just noticing the position of your legs and any pressure in the front and back of your legs. Be aware of sensations of tightness and note how they're being replaced by relaxation, just like your arms, limp and relaxed.

Note if the muscles of your stomach are contracted—such as any knotted up tension feelings—but now, replace that with loose relaxation. Let yourself sink back deeper into relaxation, not resisting it but acknowledging your controlled relaxation.

Now, focus on your face muscles around the forehead and become aware of the frowning tension being replaced by smooth relaxation, your forehead muscles becoming smooth and relaxed. Many people like to let their eyes close at this stage to enjoy deeper relaxation. Now be aware of the muscles of your jaws and any teeth-clenching tension being replaced by relaxation and deep, controlled relaxation.

Take time to enjoy your control over tension. Now form a picture in your mind, a calm picture, whether it's somewhere you know, a holiday, or trees and flowers. Through the picture, instil a deeper controlled, calm relaxation.

The more you practice this technique, the more you'll find it easier to bring on these deep, controlled feelings.

How did that feel?

Were you able to physically relax the different parts of your body? Did you feel able to move your mind onto a relaxing scene somewhere that felt calm and serene?

Sometimes, people notice that when they first try this, it feels a bit odd and they don't feel fully relaxed. Don't worry; this is perfectly normal. Like anything, it's likely to become easier with practice. And now you have practised this first form of anxiety control training, but the key is to build on this by regular and continued rehearsal.

# Chapter NINTEEN

# CURB UNHELPFUL THINKING

When suffering from depression, it is essential to build positive thinking habits. Do you ever think negatively or worry by going over things in your mind again and again? Just like other aspects of life, we can all fall into different harmful habits.

These habits of over-thinking or unhelpful thoughts can spoil your life. Some people might find themselves dwelling on the negative, for example, "*I won't enjoy it if I go*." Others criticise themselves all the time, saying things like, "*They are much better at it than me*."

Others expect the very worst to happen and jump to the worst conclusion about everything by saying things like, "*I always mess things up*."

You may also tend to focus on what other people think about you and keep worrying that others find you boring, or don't like you much at all. You may think things like, "*I'm stupid*." Should you keep saying negative things to yourself, those ideas might become a reality.

When you feel stressed out or low, you'll indulge these sorts of thoughts far more often, and they become harder to put out of mind.

These adverse patterns degrade your character and are usually not true. But when you believe these things, they worsen how you feel and affect what you do, telling you you're useless or that nobody likes you, or not to bother doing things. And if you believe them and act on them, they cause you to stop doing things. Then you withdraw from life and end up feeling even worse.

Thus, unhelpful thoughts talk you out of going out with friends, applying for that new job, speaking up at meetings, or simply doing something nice for yourself or someone else.

And of course, the less you do, the worse you feel and the worse you feel, the less you do.

You may have noticed that when you feel stressed out and low, these thoughts get supercharged and pop into your mind a lot more often.

Have you ever told anyone about how you feel when these thoughts enter your mind? If so, their answer probably consists of the words, "*Try not to think about it*."

Let's see if that works right now. Take a deep breath and try hard not to think about a white polar bear. If you're anything like me, you'll find you can think of nothing else but a white polar bear.

Or if you did manage it, you had to spend a lot of mental energy thinking about, for example, a black polar bear or a car or anything else. And that's the key lesson.

You need to find a more effective, practical way of dealing with unhelpful thoughts. Doing something about these thoughts can help boost how you feel and help you get going again.

Here's a typical example of Peggy having unhelpful thoughts.

Peggy is looking for a new job and is working on her CV. She has run out of things to say about herself in the personal statement section. She starts to slump in a chair and stares out the window. Her thoughts are reeling with messages like, "*What's the point? Loads of people will be applying. Someone else with more experience will probably get the job. I can't be bothered with this. Will I ever get a job?*"

As a result, she gives up and never sends in her application. Instead, she sits down, feeling upset and useless. These thoughts are unhelpful because they worsen how Peggy feels.

Imagine you were saying these things to yourself over and over, day in and day out, week after week. Slowly, unhelpful thoughts will grind you down and just like Peggy's case, you'll feel angry, upset, frustrated, embarrassed, guilty, sad, and lonely.

So, let's move on to what to do when this happens.

First, you need a plan. There is a type of specific plan called the Amazing Bad-Thought-Busting Programme, or ABTBP for short. First you must label the thought. For example, you might find yourself taking things to heart, beating yourself up about having a gloomy view of the future, being your own worst critic, jumping to the worst conclusions, assuming others see you in a bad light, or you might be taking responsibility for everything.

There is a pattern you might fall into time and time again. You may have already noticed that you're more prone to one or more of these thinking styles, or that you notice them more than usual when you get upset. Before you start to get too upset and caught up in these thoughts, mentally try to step back and stick a label on them. It does not have to be all your thoughts; you can start with only one.

When you label an unhelpful thought, it begins to lose its power. Soon, you will realise that it's just part of being upset. It's not the truth. It's just one of those bad thoughts.

You could even say to it, "*You're not going to get me stuck in this situation again, I'm not playing that game again.*"

Secondly, leave the thought alone.

Now you know what it is to turn your back mentally on the bad thoughts, don't challenge them or try to argue with them, just let them be. Break that cycle where the thoughts go around and around in your head. Instead, take a step back and let the thoughts 'be' instead of getting caught up in them. Choose to think about what you're doing right now. Focus on a conversation you might be having with someone else.

Sometimes, people find it helpful to mentally place the unhelpful thought in the corner of the room, like a child that's just been told to sit and be quiet. Doing so can take some practice because like celebrities and naughty kids, bad thoughts love attention. Instead, just let them be, and they will retreat eventually.

Thirdly, stand up to them. Don't be bossed about by bad thoughts. Bad thoughts—just like bullies—sound strong, but really, they're weak underneath, and they tell lies.

They say, "*You won't like doing anything,* and "*You'll fail if you try.*"

Or they say, "*You're scared,* or "*Nobody likes you.*"

These are not the truth. So, don't be bullied. If the thought says *don't,* then *do.* If the thought says *can't,* then say *can* right back at it. Call its bluff and see what happens. Stand up to the bully and you'll find what it's saying isn't true.

Fourthly, give yourself a break. Bad thoughts are how you beat yourself up when you're upset. They make you say things to yourself that you would never say to a friend. So, if you're having trouble with a bad thought, think what the person who loves you most in the whole world would say to you right now. They would disagree with the bad thoughts, wouldn't they? They would remind you you're not stupid or are bound to fail.

And—I hear you shout—what if you don't have a close friend?

Fear not! It's most likely your thought gremlins have whispered so many bad things to you over the years, that you haven't believed in yourself enough to make friends. Well, tell the gremlins to leave you alone, and go out and make a friend. It's not only possible—but probable if you really want one. So for the purpose of the exercise, imagine you have that good friend.

Go into a room by yourself and speak what your friend would say to you out loud. Say it again in a kind voice. And remember, bad thoughts tell lies, and people who love you, tell you the truth. Trust these positive thoughts and let them help you get rid of the bad thought gremlins.

And finally, look at the situation differently. Imagine what it would be like if it were a friend, not you who was experiencing the unhelpful thought. What advice would you give? Now give the same advice to yourself. Put your thoughts or worry into perspective and think of them as they are.

Will it matter so much in six months? Will you remember what the problem was? If it won't matter in six months, it's probably not that important now. How would others deal with a problem? Think about someone who seems to handle problems well and work out what they do, how they might think in that situation.

With these helpful strategies at your side, you will see that bad thoughts and depression will no longer stop you from living a life of joy, meaning, and happiness.

# Chapter TWENTY

# PUTTING DEPRESSION INTO PERSPECTIVE

Depression has many faces, two of which can either make or break a situation. The first face of depression is seen through the eyes of the person helping someone suffering from depression, which can be a friend, family member, or doctor. In the story below, we are going to look at depression through the eyes of the therapist, helping a woman named Stephanie put her situation into perspective.

The second face of depression, seen through the individual's eyes itself, delves into what Stephanie does with the help her therapist gives her. Just as in Stephanie's case, many individuals listen to those who provide help but do not take to heart what is being offered.

Only when these two faces of depression meet in the middle, form a bond, and—together—look to the future, will the perspective over depression change to something that can be overcome.

## DEPRESSION THROUGH A THERAPIST'S EYES

Stephanie came to see me after eight years of working with another therapist. She told me her story of a history of relationship failures, constantly becoming involved with men who would break her heart at around the six-month point of the relationship. She was thirty-eight years old and wanted a family. She told me that her therapist—at their last session—said to her that not all people were relationship material and maybe she was one of those people, and she should stop knocking her head up against the wall to get in an intimate, long-term relationship.

She told her to accept that her life would not be going in the direction of an intimate relationship that could lead to a family.

When I heard that, my exact response was, "Well, that is some nonsense right there!"

She was intensely interested in my reaction, and I explained that she is quite capable of being in a successful relationship and that we had to find how Stephanie herself was unconsciously doing something to herself that was causing her this difficulty with relationships and that her pattern needed to be uncovered. I was quick to add that this was not about blaming herself because none of this is intentional, but that we will discover how she blocks the very things she wants.

As I told many of my clients: *It is an inside job. So, let's start the rewiring process.*

Yes, the brain can be rewired with good therapy so that new patterns of thinking, speaking, and behaving can emerge, which could lead to very different and very positive results. I was confident Stephanie would be successful, and she felt my genuine belief in her.

We discovered she had an underlying insecurity and fear of being alone.

She had been very close to her dad who had died young; he was the parent who was more tuned in to her, and she had lost him not long after puberty. In her adult relationship life, if a man showed interest, she was hooked. She did not challenge the men early enough in the courtship to discover if they could be mature enough to handle Stephanie being herself. She would adapt to whatever behaviour they threw at her. If she got stood up on a date, she would give him another chance. If he was critical, she apologised. As long as there were times when he showed approval and affection, she would overlook the hurtful, immature behaviours. She would be in the wrong relationship for six months rather than get out of it after six dates to free her up to meet someone more suitable. She never broke up with anyone. The relationship just ended when he broke up with her, or she discovered infidelity.

Maybe six weeks into our therapy sessions, Stephanie met someone online. They had this amazing online romance, as he lived out of the country, but he told her that he would be moving back to the states and could easily settle in California, which is where she lived, and that this would happen very soon. During the winter holiday—as they had met online two months prior—he visited her and stayed two weeks. Halfway through that visit, he proposed, and she accepted. It seemed a little fast, but I felt a little better when her friend, who had referred Stephanie in the first place, assured me he seemed like a great guy and it all looked good.

He planned to go home after the holidays, sell his house in England, and they were to wed in February. Sometime in January, he called her and said that due to the economic conditions currently in Europe, he was having a harder time selling his home and they would have to delay the wedding. She was disappointed, but understood. For the next three months, she would talk, text and email daily with him, being empathic and understanding and letting him know that whenever they got married, it would be wonderful. In April, though, I got an emergency phone call from her.

Stephanie, in a panicky voice, said, "I think I blew it. I think I have made another mistake."

I replied, "I highly doubt that."

"No, I think I blew it. I constantly hear from my colleagues these questions like, "So when is the wedding?" and I say repeatedly, "I don't know yet," and it's so embarrassing. So, I told my fiancée that it was difficult at times for me and he could not believe I was complaining about how I was feeling when he was already going through enough stress with the house and the economy. Then he hung up on me, and that was two days ago.

"We usually communicate multiple times per day every day, and he's not responded to any of my texts, emails, or phone calls since. And my mother and brother both said to me that I'd better not blow another relationship."

"Wow, I'm sorry to hear that you are going through that, but firstly, your mother and brother could not have said a more incorrect and harmful thing to you. I think this is good that you are finding out some vital piece of information about your fiancée now.

"You were all about him and his feelings. As soon as you expressed your pain, you found out he was not there for you. You did not blow anything! You did what you needed to do, and now you are up against your fears and insecurities that have kept you in wrong relationships in the past. Now is the time to test him to find out if you can be hopeful or if you need to break it off entirely."

"But I don't want this to end. I love him."

"Maybe it won't end, but you need to see if he is capable of being there for you even when *he* is emotionally uncomfortable. Send him a text saying, "Your distancing behaviour is unacceptable to me. If you are going to be married to me, you need to handle when I am in some emotional pain and be there for me. Step up your game, or I am out."

"I don't know if I could send him that. I don't want to lose him," Stephanie said, close to tears.

"Does this sound familiar in your life? Do you recall responding in a very similar way in past relationships?"

"Yes, but I am scared."

"I understand. In life, there are times when you need to do the tough thing, and that is the only way to get what you want."

She didn't do it. I even said you could leave out the last sentence, and she still didn't do it. Eventually, he communicated with her, and she accepted the situation for another three months and never complained. Finally, a breakthrough was coming. During one of our sessions, I asked her if she felt she was doing anything different with him than any of the other men in her past.

She said, "No."

I said, "Look, you are a very smart woman. You are in the midst of this pattern. You are relationship material! But you will never know it unless you let me help you take more risks with this man."

She asked me what to do because it was hard to argue that her passivity and co-dependency was working in her situation. I told her to communicate with him about how hurt and disappointed she was with him in how he'd dealt with her pain in April, and that the pain was even worse now and he had to learn to be there for her, and demonstrate that to her if this relationship was to have any chance.

In those three months, we had worked through some unresolved grief of losing her father as well as self-esteem issues. I asked her to compose an email using her own words. We discussed her possible plans of action based on his response to it. She sent the email, and by the following session a week later, he had once again stopped responding to any messages and distanced himself again. This time, she followed through on what we discussed.

She promised herself and me that if there were to be no response, she would send him a goodbye email and be done. That was what she did while in the session with me, and I helped her work through her final grief.

Four months after that, she met a man from Orange County on a trip to Ireland.

He had two children from a previous marriage. She was now 39. They fell in love. She told me that some of his parenting with his children was a problem for her and that if it did not change, it could be a real problem for her. This time, without waiting, she asserted herself—saying that he needed to get into therapy because if he continued his current behaviour with his children (and ex-wife) that would be a deal-breaker for her. He agreed, went to therapy and made good progress.

They got married ten months later, and she got pregnant just after her 40th birthday and gave birth to a healthy baby girl. That was six years ago, and they have a great family life. Also, he has maintained better boundaries with his ex-wife and previous children.

From the above story, I am sure you got a little insight into what depression looks like from a therapist's perspective. Every morning when I wake up, and I look into the mirror, I whisper, "Stephanie, the face you see in the mirror is no longer that of depression alone. It is the face of triumph, determination and victory over what once held you back."

With those words of encouragement, I smile at the face in the mirror with confidence.

***

No longer do I feel depressed.

I am happy, and I have an entire lifetime to make every second count.

During my own inner struggle with depression, I discovered other tools to help control my mood. There are more ways to help myself than I realised! It was a fallacy to think that I was helpless against the onslaught of my emotions. There are occasionally things or circumstances that I cannot control, but doing what I can to fix the little things, which helps me to handle the bigger challenges so much better.  This empowerment removes the excuse of blaming others as well.

I compiled a list of questions for myself to look at when I find that I'm slipping down the hill of depression. If I address the answers quickly, I can correct myself.

- Have I eaten well today? Enough, but not too much? Too much sugar or carbohydrates?
- Have I had any exercise today, preferably outside? Something I enjoy?

- ❖ Am I busy with satisfying activities, preferably something creative? I do not consider doing chores as being creative. But it can be something like cooking a meal or even planning a meeting,.
- ❖ Have I done anything for someone else today? Again, chores do not count! It must be something for someone who is less happy than I am in some way.
- ❖ Have I had meaningful contact with people? Not empty chit chat or gossip.
- ❖ Have I laughed today?
- ❖ Is there music in my life? It can be any music.
- ❖ Is my environment organised? It can help to organise the row of shoes in front of my cupboard. Nothing obsessive!
- ❖ Have I completed a task that has been annoying me for a while? Pay a bill, organise the magazines, write an email, etc. It helps to tick things off in my diary.
- ❖ Am I overtired? Am I putting too much pressure on myself? Have I slept enough or too much?
- ❖ Have I allowed someone to manipulate or use me today?
- ❖ Did I say yes when I should have said no?
- ❖ Are there any uncertainties bothering me? Can I do something about them?
- ❖ Should I ask someone for help instead of just waiting in anxious silence?

It requires some determination to do something about this list, but it makes a very definite difference and helps me to get back on track in the right direction!

Depression is a treacherous thief. It prefers to work undercover, and likes to catch you alone, springing out at you when you were not expecting it. It churns around your mind like a storm cloud, depleting your energy and blinding you to all that is good. It will tell you to "suck it up," and then when you cannot take it any longer, it will tell you to give up.

Find courage and face your enemy. Bring in your platoon. Call for covering fire. Get somebody in that foxhole with you. Declare war! There is no shame in recognising you are surrounded by the enemy. It happens. You do not need to become a casualty when reinforcements are near. Depression will make you a prisoner or kill you if it can. It picks off the isolated, the weakened, the weary, and the silent. Dozens around you are suffering in isolation, while dozens of others are retaking the ground once occupied by despondency. And there is far too much silence. Let us change that, shall we?

Because...we are not alone.

## SOME TRUTHS ON...

### SOME TRUTHS ON...
### THE BITTER STRUGGLE OF DEPRESSED PEOPLE

You will be injured by many little, and some big, problems in your life. You should be aware of this. The world can be an evil place where people take joy in hurting others. Sometimes they hurt you unintentionally because they have no idea what your life is like, what you are going through, or they are far too overwhelmed with their own issues to care what they do to you. People will often judge you. They will try to find something negative against you rather than focusing on the positive. Judgment is hurtful, especially when people judge you negatively, which can make even a good-hearted person cynical.

The fact is that people will always behave like this. There will always be people out there who may hate you. It is impossible to satisfy everyone's expectations; people are complicated because we all think differently and we are all facing our own demons. One may have a more positive or negative opinion of an individual than he deserves. Life is filled with judgments. Have you ever been judged for your religion or where you come from, or even just for the colour of your skin?

Have you been judged for the label on your jacket or where you got your hair done?

Have you been judged for being too close to your mother, or not close enough? Or for not being environment-conscious—or for being one of those weird 'green'-obsessed people?

Let's face it, however you live your life, whatever choices you make, someone is going to disparage your decisions and lifestyle.

Being judged is humiliating, but look at the other side! If someone judges you for who or what they assume you are, without really knowing the real you, they are the ones in the wrong.

## SOME TRUTHS ON... LETTING GO OF NEGATIVE JUDGMENTS

There will always be people against you who will try to drag you down, even if you do not have any hate towards anyone. Why? Because some people are not motivated to self-improve and cannot stand seeing anyone else do well, as this reminds them of the negative feelings they have about themselves. Once you become successful in the eyes of the people who so carelessly discarded your affection and abandoned you, they may try to reach out to you and come back into your life. I have come to realise that most of the people who left me in the past probably regretted it and wished they had not done so. Some have openly admitted I was one of the best people they had known. A few even expressed remorse for what they had done to me. But sadly, it is too late for me to regain my trust in them. In the end, they lose, and I ultimately win because I am likely far better off *avoiding* having anyone in my life who disregards me and does not appreciate me for who I am.

## SOME TRUTHS ON…
## LOSS OF LOVED ONES

Sometimes, you will become sad, disappointed, or feel wholly rejected after you lose someone you have cherished. People you care about can abruptly, and too easily, disappear from your life. They block you, erase you from their thoughts, and pretend that you never existed. The problem is that humans do not appreciate the valuable diamonds they have in close relationships until they lose them.

Love–or the loss thereof–can cause you major heartache. I have had my share of this hurt. It is a horrible feeling. So many people who have cheated on me, betrayed me, or deserted me have left a lasting scar on my heart.

## SOME TRUTHS ON…
## BETTERING YOURSELF

Often, the people you keep closest to your heart will be the same ones who betray you. But, if you gave up, they would win and you would be the only one who lost. What is the purpose of your life, then? To survive, I started using my creativity, becoming someone that no one ever knew existed, someone who wants to make this world a better place. I have found this very satisfying and a way to make myself instantly happy.

## SOME TRUTHS ON…
## SEEING THE BIG PICTURE

We all experience difficult moments. One way to solve problems is to think of people who may be facing a worse time. It may seem hard but think about it; some people do not even have access to technology to read this book. Some people find themselves in war zones and have lost all their family members. At night, they shiver from fear or due to a lack of heat and nourishment. Does this image give you some perspective? Perhaps, but in our misery, we seldom take another's situation into consideration.

## SOME TRUTHS ON... WALKING FOR CALMNESS

Exercise! Walking is just one way to get rid of or reduce depression. I learned that walking long distances helped to reduce my level of depression. When I walk, I feel the stress disappearing. I usually walk at night and prefer to walk long distances. It gives me time to clear my mind and to think about life rather than concentrating on my problems.

## SOME TRUTHS ON... ORGANISING YOUR LIFE

Another method of reducing depression is to use a to-do list to help organise your life. Waking up and seeing your room in a mess emphasises the mess in your life. Completing the various cleaning tasks and putting everything in order makes you feel better and may let you view your circumstances in a more positive light. Being organised can help you feel less depressed because you have things to accomplish, things to keep you busy. And at the end of each day there is the satisfaction of checking of all the tasks you've completed. I can recommend an application called "Google Keep," which allows you to compile to-do lists, take notes, and provides a few other tools to keep you organised. Those with OCD will find it especially useful. It has certainly helped me to become less anxious.

## SOME TRUTHS ON... BEING COMPASSIONATE: HUMANS ARE IMPERFECT

Treat people better than they treat you. If someone cares for you, care for them twice as much. If someone does not care about you, the choice is yours! If someone hurts me, I still care about them, because I always believe they will realise their error and maybe change for the better one day. I am not saying I put up with being treated badly, but I tend to find a way to give people the benefit of the doubt because you do not know their circumstances.

People give up on other people, which is one of the things that still makes me very sad. But such is life, and we should always be grateful for life even when we do not understand everything. As a general rule, we should not expect that people will change, but we can hope that for their sake we do. However, we have to realize that our own happiness cannot be contingent on someone else changing or treating us the way we hope for or wish to be treated.

Oftentimes in life, people who show this sort of vision and perspective on human beings are sensitive and special individuals. You might feel frustrated at times and wonder if you should 'toughen up' and change your ways to fit in with what you perceive is the majority of people around you. Maybe the world does not understand you, but that is okay because you know the truth of who you are. Do not lose hope and most importantly, do not feel you need to change. People may relish in spreading lies to make others look bad. It is humiliating to be the object of spiteful gossip, but as long as you know who you are, it does not matter how others see you. If you learn to give the most value to what you believe about yourself, you will find that this is the ultimate source of happiness.

If you are one of those people who wastes their time listening to malicious rumours about other people, be careful to judge and even more careful to spread these tales. Even if you have all the facts—which rarely happens—you can never know or fully understand the challenges that another human being is facing. No one is perfect. Everyone makes mistakes. And remember, there are always at least two sides to every story. So, do not blindly judge someone based on what another person tells you about them. Maybe that person has hatred in his/her heart and wants to destroy their reputation, which happens a lot nowadays. If you listen to an unjustified judgment or repeat the gossip, you are just as guilty as the originator.

And even if you do have something bad to say about someone, it is almost always better not to say it. In my opinion, you should only expose a person if there is a danger present from his/her behaviour that may pose a genuine threat to another.

## SOME TRUTHS ON... WHY YOU SHOULD GET A HOBBY

Another way of reducing depression is occupying your mind with a hobby. The options are extremely varied. Some people enjoy reading, others sketch or take up other art forms such as making use of a camera to record their daily lives.

## SOME TRUTHS ON... ADDING ART TO YOUR LIFE

Art can be used to relieve stress and relax your mind and body, enabling you to clear your mind and centre your focus. It has been shown that this kind of mindfulness has meditative benefits. Colouring or drawing freely anything you like or anything that comes to mind that you want to express brings an almost instantaneous relief from anxiety and even reduces symptoms of depression. You can purchase adult colouring books online or even download colouring pages for free. It may sound a little childish to some, but don't knock what you haven't tried! It is very therapeutic and restful.

## SOME TRUTHS ON... WHY YOU SHOULDN'T OVERLOAD YOUR MIND

Overthinking can cause depression by letting you create problems that do not exist, and it usually occurs when you care about something or someone more than you should. I have been through a lot during my life. I have trusted people too easily and allowed them too close too quickly. I tried to protect them and fought for them. I deprived myself for their sake, which occurred numerous times with different people. I have a heart that is too soft, always willing to accept everyone. Until one day, they turn against me and vanish from my life.

In the past, more often than not, it was because these people had never really cared about me or weren't as close to me as they pretended. This has been a realization for me that was very difficult to face. I still find it difficult to come to terms with people's betrayal. People too easily lie to you, hurt you, and ruin your life. But life has taught me I need to love myself first and protect myself more, and that I need to be more positive about my life even if the majority of people may misunderstand me.

## SOME TRUTHS ON... MAKING YOUR GOAL A REALITY

Be careful and focus on what you want. If you have a particular goal or vision, no matter how small it is or ambitious it is, strive for it, the same way you strive to get an A+ in an exam. Life is the biggest test of all. Take it seriously and plan your future. Focus on your long-term goals, rather than on the past.

However, remember what I mentioned previously about remaining in the *here and the now*, as this is what will help you to perform your best to achieve your dreams and visions. Make the present work for you to contribute to your happiness. It is good to have and to follow a life plan but remember it may (and probably will) deviate at times. So, include the now in your life, enjoying it every day with the flexibility necessary to adjust your approach as you go.

Don't plan for the future to the detriment of living in and relishing the present, since that is obsessive and may even prove futile!

Learn to enjoy the now and integrate into each week time to plan for the future, but without letting it dominate everything you do. There is much balance required when making your goals a reality, but you will find that when you find the right rhythm, you will see the results you envision.

## SOME TRUTHS ON....
## COPING WITH DECEPTION

In life, you will meet various types of people, and sadly, many of them will be insincere, fake, or will seek to take advantage of you and not care about you.

I always try to help all people and to create amicable relationships with everyone. I have had to learn to accept that not everyone is going to like me or treat me with the same consideration. Sometimes you will help people who will repay you with unkindness, deceit, and hurt. These factors are close to impossible to control in life. Look at life as a test. Sometimes those tests will come through trials and struggles with the people you consider closest to you. You may feel as if you have lost everything by losing just one immensely cherished person.

From time to time, people may abandon you and try to make it seem as if it is your fault. But it is their problem. They may falsely accuse you or blame you for something to make leaving you easier on them, whether they leave you physically or abandon you emotionally. In some cases, you may learn the truth later eventually. Oftentimes, people are afraid or do not know how to tell you that their feelings towards you have changed. So instead, they hurt you. The hurt may not be intentional or deserved, but they go ahead and do it anyway.

The saddest part is that people will not always reciprocate the kindnesses you show them. Sometimes, if you care about and value someone too much, they will take advantage of you, or turn on you and make you look like you are the bad person. Be careful who you trust; the people you love may not always feel the same about you. To me, the worst loss is when someone I care about and have invested my affection in, moves on.

Life is an unceasing series of tests. How will you handle these challenges?

Use the opportunity before it is too late. You and I do not know when we will leave this planet, this existence. Once you die, the opportunity to rectify the many things you wished you could change in this lifetime ends. So, do not keep delaying doing well in life. Plan your new improved self. Start working on it today. Do not give up.

## SOME TRUTHS ON...
## WHY YOU NEED A REALITY CHECK

We all need someone who is there for us, who understands us, and especially someone we highly and value in our lives. But from time to time, that person is not available or simply chooses not to be there for us, and we have to accept whoever we have around us.

If you feel you need to talk to that certain special person in your life, what do you do if they will not allow you to talk to them? You end up living your own life, trying to figure it out all by yourself. Accept the people who do appreciate you, and those who value you unreservedly.

We cannot always make everyone in our lives—even the ones we love dearly—happy. First of all, when it comes to adult relationships, it is not anyone's job to make someone else happy. Happiness is our own personal responsibility; true happiness, that is. And it is not because we do not care about those around us enough to make an effort to make them happy, but rather because happiness is a personal endeavour and life journey related to our own self-development.

To be able to understand what each of us is going through, we have to help one another, love one other, and do our utmost not to harm each another. At least, this should be the ideal to strive for.

Sometimes, people who mean a lot to you may not understand you and choose to believe that whatever you do is always against them, even if it is not true. So, what do you do in such a scenario? You can make an effort to help them understand your true intentions, but accept that not everyone will. Everyone has his or her own type of depression. Some have problems related to depression, while other problems are not necessarily related to this affliction. You can try to make them see you for who you are, but not everyone is going to be satisfied with your explanations or with what you do. Accept this as part of life.

Not everyone is going to accept you, which is another thing that may be hard to live with. The most important thing is that YOU know your intentions are good, although people may misinterpret them. Maybe they do not understand what you are doing or why you are doing it. Maybe they do not understand you. Maybe, in the future, one day they will want to get to know and understand you better. Maybe, but nothing is certain. We only have control over our own actions, decisions, and behavours.

If someone appreciates you, they will take the time and exert the effort to understand you. If people care about you, they will not want to lose you or leave you. They will want to be with you and be willing to fight for you.

## SOME TRUTHS ON... STAYING POSITIVE

Depression is not something you can "get over." The longer you are immersed in this darkness, the more difficult it becomes to get out. Even when you think that you have vanquished the monster, it can return and drag you back into the depths of despair. The only way to conquer it is to get back up when you stumble, and to keep fighting.

Depression can be very dangerous, both mentally and physically. You will end up doing things you do not want to do.

Always remember it is not your fault if people want to leave you, especially if you have not done something to hurt them intentionally. It is their decision, and ultimately, their loss, not yours. They may come back to you after a month or a year, and you may have changed by that time, leaving them feeling the same way you had previously felt about them. Do not hurt one another. If you are the type of person who leaves others easily, think about the misery you cause and work on fixing this personality trait.

## SOME TRUTHS ON... BEING PRODUCTIVE

Different people have different things they do to occupy themselves. Being productive prevents you from wasting your time thinking about problems that you cannot solve, or that will take a lot of time for you to solve with insufficient gain afterwards. There are various ways to become productive and to accomplish tasks. By completing tasks, you become free, and that will give you more time to focus on the bigger issues. Always try to complete your routine tasks before you try to solve the big problems—unless, of course, the problem will not allow you to concentrate on the task at hand.

## SOME TRUTHS ON... THE SAFETY ZONE

The biggest initial need for someone in the grip of depression is to have a safety zone, whuch usually consists of someone in whom you can confide without feeling judged, exposed, ridiculed, or misunderstood. This person may be a professional or initially a spouse, friend or family member. It is often easier to seek professional help once you feel safe and able to confide your deepest feelings and fears to someone.

It helps immensely to understand that chronic depression is a disease. There is no shame in catching the flu, no threat to one's reputation in having Lyme disease. Neither is there shame in having a mental disease like depression. Doctors, therapies and medicines are there for a reason—

to fix what ails us, whether it is in our skin, our blood, our lungs, or our psyche.

I have a friend who has a big scar on his bald head. He needed brain surgery, a medical intervention in his brain to save his life. He will joke about it, just as I sometimes joke about needing my happy pill each day. I'm very glad he's alive, and (I think) he feels the same about me. In both cases, someone outside of ourselves had to see the problem and provide the fix.

Be aware that often, the depressed person whom you love cannot see clearly at all. It is like walking around with dark glasses in a dimly-lit room. The denial is sometimes quite subconscious. A darkened world becomes their normality.

It is very tempting to want to shake a depressed person by the shoulders and yell, "*Just snap out of it, will you*?"

That is about as useful as slapping me across the face and saying, "*Just see clearly, will you*?"

I am quite depressed, and I cannot see clearly until the right glasses are prescribed and worn.

Is it difficult to put away the coping mechanisms and to admit, "*I have a problem.*"

It seems like a huge risk when you are still living under dark clouds. That is why you need a safe place. What is truly risky is living under dark clouds and hoping they will go away. My experience has been that people are relieved, encouraged, and happy to know that I am human and that I'm getting better. And, I can then try, if only for the reason that I am able to help others instead of staying locked up and paralysed in my dark corner.

What if you have a friend or family member you believe is depressed, and who cannot seem to talk about it? I can't give professional clinical advice, but I will tell you the kinds of questions that, lovingly asked, helped me to start talking.

*How are you doing?*

*No, how are you really doing?* (In private of course).

Do not settle for the "*just fine*" brush-off.

*"You look a bit down. Is there something you would like to talk about for a few minutes? I'm ready to listen."*

Corner the person with an observation and an offer, otherwise they'll feel like no-one else should be sharing their burden.

*Is there anything specific I can pray about for you, other than the usual same-old?* That's said with a smile, and it's an invitation to unburden which just might be taken.

*"I am having some problems."*

Yes! I really do mean that you share the fact your life is also problematic. Of course, just allude to it and don't forget the aim here is *to get your friend to talk about their concerns*; try not to ramble on about yourself, leaving no time or emotional energy for their issue.

They may not have the residual energy to cope with their own scenario if they have to counsel you on yours first. However, a sense of togetherness is good, and this is what you seek to create in saying you have a problem. We all have problems to address, but frequently the depressed person feels isolated. One of the things that can be very therapeutic for someone under the clouds weighed down by this wretchedness is helping someone else out, opening the door for them to share their burdens. Depending on the relationship, this next suggestion may or may not be appropriate.

However, in the right setting, the simple act of hugging someone who is hurting can begin to open the floodgates. Get in a safety zone. *Be* a safety zone. Depression wants to isolate. Do not allow it to happen.

## SOME TRUTHS ON... THE PATH TO RECOVERY

It would be nice to say that waving a magic wand could make depression go away. However, ingrained patterns of thoughts and feelings, especially if fuelled by brain chemistry and past traumas, take time to unwind. It is okay to be "recovering." While there is often a (real or perceived) stigma about admitting to having certain conditions, what I have found is that people are very receptive—and often relieved—to find a fellow traveller. The silence is what prolongs the disease and fuels its intensity. It is far riskier to go on suffering alone than to seek help and companionship.

Some medical approaches may be more, or less, effective depending on the individual. It could be that you will be stuck with an emotional limp for the rest of your days. Whatever the case, would you please drop the mask and join many sufferers who are limping their way forward? We need your strength, your gifts, and your insights, and you are welcome to borrow ours. Yes, it would be so nice to have it all together. However, if, like me, you cannot accomplish that, let us settle for reality and humanity. But please, whatever you do—do not give up!

# INDEX

## A



## B



## C

## D



## E



## F



## G

## H



## I



## J



## K



## L

## M



## N



## O



## P

## T



## W



## Y

Made in the USA
Coppell, TX
05 November 2026

11315641R00102